Questions & Answers
on Nervous System Related Disorders

Seventy-Seven Thought-Provoking Q & As!

By: James M. Lowrance © 2010

2

TABLE OF SECTIONS:

3

INTRODUCTION:

There are <u>many health disorders</u> that are related to the
functioning of the nervous system, which is comprised
of sensory, motor and autonomic nerves. The "Involuntary
Nervous System", is <u>especially vulnerable to imbalances</u>
within it that can occur due to hormone imbalances,
vitamin deficiencies, emotional and mental disorders and
nervous system, spinal cord and brain abnormalities.

In this approximately 23,000 word book, I have compiled
a number of responses I made to fellow patients on patient
support forums, who were experiencing **nervous system
related health disorders**, such as peripheral neuropathies,
myopathies (neuromuscular problems) and nervous
system diseases. These responses, which are presented as
<u>well-informed layperson opinions</u>, include my personal
experiences with nervous system symptoms as related to
my thyroid disease, peripheral neuropathies, myopathy,
Mitral Valve Prolapse Syndrome and vitamin deficiency
diagnoses.

An important aspect of online symptom searches that I
mention in several opinions I include in this book are on
the subject of "cyberchondria" (also called "surf diagnosis
induced anxiety") , **a serious anxiety reaction** that can
occur in patients who do not understand the importance of
<u>balanced medical searches</u>, on reputable online sources.

It is my hope that these 77 short, individual opinion-posts
(averaging approximately 300 words each) will prove to
be beneficial to the readers of them. – Jim Lowrance

4

NOTE: Proper diagnosis and treatments for health disorders of <u>any kind</u> must always be obtained through qualified, medical professionals.

SECTION ONE:
Questions and Answers/Opinions 1 through 20

Q & A: OPINION ONE

Muscle Twitching - Sign of a Dreaded Disease?

Many medical sites list "muscle twitching" as a symptom of peripheral neuropathy, among other things, including "stress and anxiety" that can cause muscle twitches.

QUOTE - from New York Presbyterian Hospital:

"Peripheral neuropathy produces symptoms such as weakness, muscle cramps, twitching, pain, numbness, burning, and tingling (often in the feet and hands)."

With common health problems such as diabetes (many times undiagnosed), nerve entrapment, nutritional deficiencies and at least 25% of cases being "idiopathic" (no detectable cause), the jump should not be made, in believing that combinations of symptoms such weakness and muscle pain or twitching with tingling - automatically indicates something like ALS (a fatal motor neuron disease). One should rather recognize the fact that this disorder, among many others needs to be checked-for as an overall medical evaluation. Certainly this type of jumping to worst-case–scenario conclusions doesn't happen frequently but often-enough to contribute to the growth of the "cyberchondria" (health anxiety) problem that affects up to 5% of the population according to some sources.

This actually inspired research studies by Microsoft Research Corporation in regard to the growing cyberchondria problem.

Most medical people and layperson members of forums and websites do give better-perspective type answer to patients inquiring online about their neurological symptoms but I have seen some replies to posts by those fearing a terminal disease, to be answered with insensitivity. In fact I saw a post by someone who had muscle twitching in one limb, followed by a reply made to them that was to the effect: *"that type symptom is concerning for ALS."* Yet if you go to e-health forums regarding muscle twitches and anxiety (MedHelp is my favorite medical forum), people by the hundreds are experiencing muscle twitches, anywhere from that found in one limb to those that occur body-wide.

If one wanted to go this far, they could even say that ALS or any other terminal illness is a possibility in ANYONE, regardless of symptoms or even **if they have no symptoms at all** (also true of other disease such as cancer). That would actually be a true statement as well but it certainly lacks perspective and deserves a balanced answer, more properly perspected for the sake of those searching online, in regard to their concerning symptoms.

<u>Q & A: OPINION TWO</u>

Sensory and Motor Peripheral Neuropathies

I have found through balanced, online medical search - this time for information in regard to the function of sensory versus motor and autonomic nerves that "peripheral neuropathies" involving sensory nerves do cause muscle weakness. Examples: carpal tunnel syndrome, tarsal tunnel syndrome, sural neuropathy, tibial neuropathy, peronial neuropathy, median neuropathy, etc...... These types can affect both sensory and motor nerves to muscles and may remain isolated or may affect several areas of the body (polyneuropathy) but still not be in the neuromuscular, degenerative disease category.

The ones listed above having to do with the feet, ankles and upper legs, can cause muscle weakness in these areas, lack of muscle control in them and even muscle atrophy (wasting) in severe cases and this would be a result of the peripheral neuropathy (diabetes being a common cause). The medical sources that give information on these nerve related disorders also mention "foot drop" and limb deformity from these affected nerves in some cases.

The same is true of the nerves listed above that affect the hand and upper-arm. I in-fact just spoke to a man a weeks ago (at the time of this writing), who used to be a carpenter but he began suffering "carpal tunnel syndrome" in his hands and wrists and he had to change occupations because he was literally losing use of his hands.

He told me that he could barely hold-up a cup of coffee due to the weakness and shaking in them. Fortunately, his resolved without nerve surgery.

Patients who begin experiencing nerve or muscle problems in their limb(s) should understand that peripheral neuropathies are very common and that qualified doctors can diagnose the types affecting a patient (over 100 types exist) and the causes of them, so that proper treatment(s) can be administered.

Q & A: OPINION THREE

Avoiding Contributing to the Cyberchondria Trend

I actually mention some of the things that follow in the post (converted to article) below, in other recent articles but with "cyberchondria" becoming an increasingly serious problem; I feel some of these points should be made, as an ongoing reminder, to keep a better balance on forums and online searches. ---

I'm one of MANY patients, found to have peripheral neuropathy symptoms (estimates - 20,000,000 Americans) and because of the rare possibility of ALS (Amyotrophic Lateral Sclerosis – "Lou Gehrig's Disease") being a cause via search engine reading, I began the neurotic search for confirmation against having it or another neuromuscular degenerative disease.

Even after I started this trend and my neurologist told me at least twice with **firm conviction**, that neither my symptoms nor my EMG - nerve conduction studies pointed to ALS, I still sought secondary confirmation through forums and more online search etc... Also, my having been found deficient in two major vitamins (D and E) and insufficient in B12, already gave me an obvious cause of my peripheral neuropathy, as does my autoimmune thyroid disease. I also have the burning, stabbing and tingling sensations (sensory symptoms) not typical of motor neuron disease (MND) but more-so of typical peripheral neuropathy (far more common).

Yes, ALS is a real disease, absolutely and though still rare, is more common than previously discovered. God bless those who have this life-altering and fatal disease and those that are less catastrophic but still life changing, such as other types of MND and MS (Multiple Sclerosis).

With this said, I, Jim Lowrance -- the writer of this article, have seen a trend in which statements are made online, to the effect on sites and forums: *"muscle weakness can mean you have a neuromuscular degenerative disease"* or that *"muscle twitching"* can mean this. While this statement is true, it could be balanced a bit more by adding statements to the effect that many things can cause these and other symptoms, yes, even muscle atrophy (wasting) that are not one of these diseases (i.e. metabolic myopathies, hyperthyroidism, diabetes, nutritional deficiencies, etc...).

Giving someone a worse-case-scenario **right off the bat**, when they are seeking some general information about their symptoms, can begin a trend in their search that will cause them a great deal of anguish. I do not believe it hurts to mention these severe diseases that cause symptoms in the early onset of them that are similar to those that are much less-severe, as long as the reader understands that such mentions are by no means a suggestion that they have such an illness. They should also understand that an in-person medical evaluation, by a qualified doctor is the only way to be definitively diagnosed and to rule-out the more serious but less-common possibilities.

Q & A: OPINION FOUR

POTS and CFS - Symptom Similarities

CFS (Chronic Fatigue Syndrome) and POTS (Postural Orthostatic Tachycardia Syndrome), the second one being a condition of imbalanced involuntary nervous system symptoms (dysautonomia), are two disorders that have often been confused with each other and some people who've been diagnosed with one actually have the other. This is one of those unfortunate things that happens in medical practice, especially when doctors do not recognize the existence of one medical condition or the other. Strangely, some doctors recognize neither of them and I know this first-hand by asking some licensed physicians I have been-to.

Some admitted that they had never even heard of POTS or dysautonomia but most knew about CFS, they just didn't feel it was a real illness. Apparently they haven't read the U.S. National Institutes of Health pages on CFS, which not only gives statistics on CFS but clearly stated diagnostic criteria for it as well.

I Jim Lowrance, the writer of this article, believed from 2003 to year (2010) that I had comorbid CFS to my autoimmune thyroid disease, until 2 vitamin deficiencies (E and D) were found and an insufficient B12 level (lower-normal). I now believe these are largely responsible for my neuro-type symptoms but I also believe my dysautonomic symptoms would meet the criteria for POTS (i.e. drop in blood pressure upon standing and elevation of heart rate). CFS in medical research studies has revealed orthostatic hypotension as a common feature of it, which shows how closely related these conditions are.

One thing that will comfort one who suspects they may have one of these illnesses, as they go through the process of elimination and the diagnosis of what is actually affecting them, is that other serious disorders are also being ruled out during the diagnostic process. Not that I'm placing POTS or CFS in the non-serious category because they can be life disrupting and seriously affect quality of life but treatments can help a great deal with symptoms and they are not typically life-threatening. Some people actually see full recovery from CFS in 2 to 5 years or longer.

I personally know 2 people who fully recovered from the illness and no longer experience its symptoms at all. Full recovery may not be common, but gives patients something to place hope in as they undergo their treatments.

Q & A: OPINION FIVE

What causes Sensory Nerve Sensations in the Legs?

This article is derived from a reply I, Jim Lowrance, made to someone asking about "goose pimple" type sensations occurring on their lower legs, which would likely be a mild type of peripheral neuropathy involving sensory nerves as I related in my reply which follows:

"I've been found to have some low-normal and slightly below normal EMG (electromyography) readings associated with neuropathy symptoms I also experience. I found similarity to those you describe with my occasional flare of this type symptom. Mine occurs usually on the back of my left calf and feels like a small wave of goose pimples, like when you hear a song that give you chills - some people even used to say that U.S. President – Barack Obama, gave them chills that ran up their legs (LOL). Mine also feels at times, a bit like something is touching my legs, other than my pant legs... an interesting but strange symptom!

When you get that type symptom it is usually from a **sensory nerve** and it can be due to them being impinged (pinched) or injured. A damaged **motor nerve** causes lack of coordination and fatigue in the muscle. With peripheral neuropathies, one or both types of nerves can be affected. Anxiety can aggravate neuropathy type problems but it isn't a direct cause of them. If it's not actually a problem in nerves but just an anxiety symptom, the nerves would not be injured or in need of repair/treatment. That would mean it's "psychosomatic" but in most cases, peripheral neuropathy causes those type problems and is very common (affecting approximately 20-million people in the U.S. alone).

A doctor of neurology would be able to tell you more about why the symptom is happening.

Q & A: OPINION SIX

Finding a Compassionate Doctor who Listens

The following article was derived from forum replies I made to a fellow patient, who like many others, was first given the "emotional diagnosis" for physical symptoms they knew for a fact to be caused by a medical, rather than an emotions-only condition. I added suggestions, as to what type tests they might need ordered for further evaluation and I also added quotes by medical sources, in regard to "doctor burn-out" and "patient-doctor communication" issues. ---

You may need even more blood tests because I can assure you they haven't covered every possibility yet. There are things such as vitamin levels for example that can have a profound affect when they become deficient (D, E, B6 and B12). They may just simply need to keep looking until they find the cause and sometimes this is a long process of elimination.

The depression diagnosis your doctor originally resorted-to, is reported by so many patients who were later found to have true medical problems (I'm one of them) that it reveals a disturbing trend. I must balance that by saying there are fabulous doctors who do take more interest, time and care for difficult cases and if you get any inkling that one is not doing so, in light of your symptoms that have been life-altering for you, I would seek a referral to another specialist.

Used-to, it was taboo to point out less-than-adequate doctors, however, even the U.S. National Institutes of Health and other medical groups are starting to warn about doctor burn-out, etc... and are also beginning to educate the public to look for signs of this. I've had people doubt me on this and I've referred them to the sources for this and they are amazed at how this type thing is somewhat in denial by most of the public and especially by some in the medical community.

Some doctors do not listen to their patients or they listen selectively, so that they only hear part of what they are saying.

I have actually left doctors for that reason, to find ones willing to listen and not keep me on a time clock. At the same time, I'm respectful of their time and do not feel I've ever taken advantage of it (despite how detailed I sometimes am on forum posts).

Here are two quotes from medical organizations regarding doctor-patient communication:

The National Academy of Medicine: *"Establishing and maintaining strong partnerships between health care providers and patients is crucial to reducing medical errors."*

Mack Lipkin MD, founding president of the American Academy on Physician and Patient: *"An activated patient who asks questions and negotiates with the doctor has better outcomes ...The most important predictor of compliance is trust in the doctor; that begins with communication."*

I hope your current doctor(s) have also tested other hormone levels, like your adrenal and sex ones. I've known people who had symptoms that would not seem to be related to these type things but it ends up being their problem. My suspicion is that they have tested these already or are planning to, plus many other things likely yet to be tested, to further evaluate your symptoms.

Q & A: OPINION SEVEN

My Medical Forum Inquiry Regarding Vitamin E Deficiency

When I was found to have vitamin E deficiency in June of 2010, I posted questions regarding the deficiency on a reputable medical forum. Since posting the question, I was able to receive answers to my questions and I am now on a maintenance dose of vitamin E that is 200IU per day. I believed for many years that my unresolved symptoms were thyroid disease related or from a comorbid condition such as Chronic Fatigue Syndrome. ---

"I've sought an answer to this question on other website forums but so far, due to the rarity of vitamin E deficiency, I have so-far not received any answers. I was found to be vitamin E deficient with a reading of "0.4 ng/dL", which is less than a half point, with normal value range at Quest being "3.0 to 16.0". My doctor is having me take 400 IU of E supplementation and after only three weeks on it, my level went up to about 13.0 - the higher part of the normal range, so he thought I should cut back to a replacement dose of only 50 IU but he admits he is not very familiar with E deficiency and not completely sure about this dosage.

My question is kind of multi-part but I would appreciate any opinion you have on any of it.

MY OWN QUESTION SPECIFICALLY: Do you know how long supplementation takes, to see neuropathy symptoms caused by E deficiency to resolve and was my 0.4 result indicative of 'severe deficiency' and lastly, is it typical to see a deficient level rise to a higher normal level so quickly?

I was also found deficient in D and low-normal in B12 and I definitely don't believe the E result was a lab fluke due to the testing procedure for vitamins being so highly specialized.

My symptoms: peripheral neuropathy and muscle weakness/myopathy, that goes back at least 7 years and more likely 10 years but no muscle atrophy/shrinkage as yet."

(Note: Due to the rarity of vitamin E deficiency, I did not receive an answer to this forum inquiry however; my doctors have since researched the condition and have provided me better answers and a specific treatment regimen -- being 200IU vitamin E maintenance dose daily, which followed the higher, short-term replacement dose for the deficiency.)

Q & A: OPINION EIGHT

Can Elevated Cortisol Indicate Adrenal Fatigue?

This article is derived from replies I made to forum posts a fellow-patient made in regard to their findings of having elevated cortisol levels.

A general MRI (Magnetic Resonance Imaging test) they had performed, was clear - indicating that the cortisol imbalance was not a brain-gland problem (dysfunction of master endocrine glands). ---

(Note: The adrenal glands are also endocrine organs (hormone producing) that are regulated by the INS-Involuntary Nervous System.)

"That elevated cortisol in both blood and urinary measure, sounds like an important lead to me because it might indicate a trend toward "Cushing's disease" (abnormally high adrenal cortisol levels), which in many cases is treated with a cortisol-inhibiting drug. It could be that this has been detected early because some people experience fatigue and muscle weakness as the first symptoms, as you have described experiencing.

Adrenal fatigue (mild adrenal insufficiency) can cause high cortisol as well, in *the alarm phase* of it, before a progressive drop in it begins to happen but with this sub-clinical type adrenal dysfunction/insufficiency, the cortisol usually fluctuates within the normal values range or just slightly outside of it. With your 24 hour random urinary cortisol being high, that means it averages high rather than just spiking at times and is why the urinary measure is the test most often used to detect Cushings disease.

They may next want to take an MRI of your pituitary gland and an endocrinologist-Dr. would definitely be who you need a referral-to, for more complete evaluation of it.

If they were not specifically trying to rule-out or confirm a pituitary gland problem in your initial MRI, they may have been conducting more of a general MRI and it may take a highly qualified endocrinologist to perform a more specific one. In addition to that, I can guarantee you they have more blood work that has yet to be done that might also still hold answers.

You would be amazed at how many things there are that can be checked for, many of them having to do with nutritional deficiencies that one would never suspect they have that can be in the mineral, vitamin, proteins and electrolyte categories.

Both my mother and my sister for example, had episodes of **passing out** at different times, with no explanation. Amazingly, with my mother, she was found to have low potassium and with my sister it was low sodium. In fact the doctor that found my sister's low sodium said it was so bottomed-out, that it was "undetectable" and he was amazed that she was still functioning. Over time, your doctor(s) will zero-in on the cause of your symptoms."

Q & A: OPINION NINE

My Experience with Nutritional Deficiencies

I have some peripheral neuropathies that seemingly also involve motor nerves because I have some clumsiness in my hands and legs at times and some muscle-weakness, in addition to sensory nerve type problems of aching, stabbing and hot pins/needles sensations.

My neurologist had the forethought to order vitamins I had yet to be tested, including E and B6. My E was very deficient, which all by itself can account for my neuropathies. Even so, he is making sure to rule out other contributing factors. He has ran across E deficiency, so rarely, that he was not totally sure what dose I needed to replace my low levels and then afterward, what dose to maintain my E levels. This is why I've posted this as a question on some medical forums - at the same time adding other aspects to my questions to forum experts.

With my having 2 vitamin deficiencies (E and D) and low-normal B12 (all now treated), he saw a trend toward nutritional problems, so he then ordered me an "L-Carninitine" level because this one can cause neuro-symptoms when low as well (results on this one were normal). I mention my case, to give example of the process of testing more things as a doctors goes along with the diagnostic process. It seems to take *as slow as an itch* and I too become impatient at times with the process but all we can do is to be patient, learn as much as we can as we go along and ask questions - including that you can ask on quality medical forums. I suppose that's where the term "patient" comes from because we have to go through such a drawn-out process at times for diagnosis and treatment to be determined.

Q & A: OPINION TEN

Cyberchondria - The Very Real Anxiety Disorder

(Note: the anxiety mechanism called "the fight or flight response", is an aspect of the "sympathetic nervous system" that can activate at <u>inappropriate times</u>, which is where the term "anxiety disorder" is derived from.)

I recently shared a post on a forum in attempt to give comfort to those, who through online search have come across worse-case scenarios for their symptoms, whether it occurs on a forum or even on the most reputable medical information websites. I stated in the post that I believe with absolute conviction that the perspective I gave in regard to researching medical and health information *responsibly and in-balance*, needs added from time-to-time as a reminder on online patient-support resources. I also specifically praised the fact that excellent support and information forums do exist and I personally love them.

I had a friend who committed suicide because he believed he had cancer developing in his leg. It first of all shocked me beyond belief but it also made me crumble for a while emotionally because I had opportunity (even felt impressed to do so) to comfort him in the fact that he should not fear the worst.

I also used to be a moderator of a thyroid disease forum and a lady who was posting there for her daughter, at one point, let the members know there, that her daughter committed suicide due to severe anxiety symptoms from Graves' disease.

She believed after many months of struggle that her case was not treatable and she simply could not take the pressure. This broke my heart beyond description.

If you do a search on "cyberchondria" (films on the subject are available on YouTube), it will give you a better sense of how serious the phobia from imbalanced information from online symptom-searches can be. I'll give one more example; I read a thread posted by a man who was experiencing muscle twitching in one leg but he reported no muscle weakness or atrophy and the response he received was *"That is concerning for ALS"*. As you know, ALS is a 100% fatal disease and most patients succumb to it in 2 to 3 years, with only a few going as long as 10 or even longer (rare). Can you imagine the **potential anguish** that type of information might place on such an individual?

I'm a "patient advocate" and I have corresponded with 1,000s of patients since 2004 and I'm an author of many medical eBook titles, all found on Amazon. I learned about trends over the years and one that has proven to be detrimental to the emotional health of some patients, has been the cyberchonria issue. Despite this, I am 100% for self-education **in-balance** and support forums and I always will be but I do believe there should be an ongoing awareness (reminders) of the possibility that some patients may be at risk for developing cyberchondria and we who post online certainly do not want to contribute to this very real anxiety disorder.

Finally, Microsoft conducted a study Re: "cyberchondria", led by a computer scientist with a medical degree, here is quote by him that is also found on the New York Times site:

"People tend to look at just the first couple results," Mr. Horvitz said. "If they find 'brain tumor' or 'A.L.S.,' that's their launching point."

It may seem at a first glance of this phenomenon, that this is a rare happening but it is affecting an estimated "5%" of the population (per "Associated Content Website"), which is huge. This is why occasional reference/warning to it should be given in my opinion.

Q & A: OPINION ELEVEN

Medical Forums - A Place of Fear or Support?

Telling someone with muscle twitches and/or weakness in their body or muscles, something to the effect of *"Oh my, you need to be evaluated for ALS* (a fatal type of motor neuron disease) *because those are the symptoms it can present with"* or *"you could very well be suffering from Multiple sclerosis"* is tantamount to telling someone with stomach pain, that they might very well have cancer. Would cancer be a possibility in the case of stomach pain? Of course it would (so would IBS that affects 15 million Americans) in-fact people with **no symptoms at all** are at the same risk for cancer as anyone else.

This is also true people who serve in the medical community. Cancer in-fact can cause neuropathy symptoms as well and the general risk for cancer is <u>ten times</u> that of ALS.

Certainly a definitive diagnosis must come through a qualified medical professional but there is also nothing wrong with basically educating one's self online in regard possibilities for medical symptoms, *as long as one searches responsibly*, balancing the information they find, <u>properly</u>.

If you do a search on *"anxiety stress muscle twitches"*, people by the 1,000s, online are attesting to having "Benign Fasciculation Syndrome", a <u>disturbing but not harmful</u> condition of muscle twitching and mild spasms and many were terrified they had ALS due to medical searches they conducted online. Other forums such as ones on Generalized Anxiety Disorder and muscle spasms reveal the **same thing** and many of these people attest to muscle weakness as well. One writer for the Associated Content website, has actually begun trying to balance the "muscle twitches" issue in a series of articles he began writing after his own ALS neurosis, was triggered by online search.

I had a doctor on a neurology forum, give me a wonderful, balanced answer to my questions about my own neuro-type symptoms and medical tests.

I had to find a cause of these, in-fact his answer is what inspired me in regard to *balanced answers* people need to hear (ones with better perspective) when they are concerned about symptoms they are having, whether from medical people or laypersons (including fellow patients). It's not wrong to point out the "possibility" of terminal illnesses, when someone posts on a forum for example, in regard to their symptoms, as long as you <u>do not</u> leave them with the impression that the most severe and rarest type diseases are the only possibilities that might be affecting them.

Note: "Cyberchondria" is also referred to as "surf-diagnosis" and "availability bias" but despite this fact, good online medical forums are **extremely valuable** for support and information.

Q & A: OPINION TWELVE

Some Medical Websites that Contribute to "Cyberchondria"

I know for a fact that my opinion regarding *"some information"* on forums and websites is not balanced at times and causes *unnecessary fears and phobias* in some readers, is not my opinion alone. You can in fact, find a great deal of information on this phenomenon by using "cyberchonria" as a search term. For example: I did a search on "muscle weakness and twitching" and came across huge numbers of sites referencing ALS.

This is a rapidly progressing "motor neuron disease", that is fatal in 100% of cases. It certainly is **a real disease**, as are other terminal illnesses but information on these needs to be balanced with facts of how common they are in relation to other disorders that cause similar or identical symptoms.

ALS for example affects an estimated 20,000 people in the U.S. (120,000 worldwide) but the more common peripheral neuropathies, of which there are **over 100 types**, affect an estimated 20,000,000 people in the U.S. alone (1,000 times as many) and these can all potentially present with symptoms similar to MND (motor neuron disease) and MS (Multiple Sclerosis), including muscle weakness (i.e. carpal and tarsal tunnel). Does this mean people SHOULD NOT be told about the possibility of having one of these diseases? **Of course not** – they should be told but, that possibility should be given to them in-balance and with some perspective in regard to the more common illnesses that cause same-symptoms. This can help offset some of the intense fears people may develop who are conducting online searches in regard to their symptoms.

Q & A: OPINION THIRTEEN

My Neurologist's Explanation Re: Benign Fasciculations

I had a follow up visit with my neurologist on the 27th of July, 2010. As a process of diagnosing and ruling out suspected causes of my myopathy (muscle weakness) and neuropathy type symptoms, he's having further muscle-related tests done because he feels if there is a direct muscle cause, it would likely be a *"metabolic myopathy"*. One of the tests will be to further rule out Myasthenia Gravis (autoimmune muscle disease). He leans toward this being an *"axonal peripheral neuropathy"* and he assured me that neither my blood tests nor my EMG/NCS (nerve studies) indicate motor neuron disease and specifically he said that my clinical picture does not pose a suspicion for ALS.

I also learned an important fact by him, in-that muscle twitches which are very commonly "benign fasciculations", are usually stress/anxiety related and don't present the same as those that occur with MNDs. He also pointed out that they do not occur before significant **muscle atrophy** has first taken place. I have no atrophy in any muscles, even with 10 years of noticeable muscle weakness that occurs with strenuous use of them and my muscle twitches are intermittent (sometimes months or years between) and can occur even in the trunk of my body, on my scalp, etc...

I have suffered anxiety since my teens but it is well-controlled for the-most-part and is the likely cause of my BFS (Benign Fasciculation Syndrome).

I'll likely have several months of testing, since only one test can usually be done per month (I've yet to understand why more tests cannot be done in combination and with less time between them), which may include *nerve/muscle biopsy* and *spinal tap* (Lumbar puncture).

Q & A: OPINION FOURTEEN

My Symptoms of Imbalanced – Involuntary Nervous System

This article is derived from a forum post I made in reply to someone asking me, if I had received a definitive diagnosis of "dysautonomia" (involuntary nervous system imbalance). ---

No, I haven't been diagnosed as yet, only the past diagnoses of Hashimoto's thyroiditis, with hypothyroidism and vitamin deficiencies (D, E and B12). Otherwise my only other diagnosis was *non-alcoholic fatty liver* (I'm a moderately overweight middle-age male). One reason I feel strongly that dysautonomia (imbalance in my nervous system) has a part in this, is the fact of my having *orthostatic hypotension* - dizziness upon first standing, from a temporary drop in blood pressure (since my teens), which though not severe, seems to have roots in **my fatigue**.

I may yet request an echocardiogram (sound wave imaging of my heart) - my mother has Mitral Valve Prolapse (common heart murmur) with mild regurgitation - she is now age-74.

I have considered MS - *Multiple Sclerosis* as a possibility for my muscle fatigue however, I had a clear MRI less than 3 years ago and my neurologist re-reviewed it when I went to him recently and he said **it was clear** as well. When I had the MRI done, I had the same symptoms I have now with exception of my having a bit more *sensory type symptoms now* - occasional hot needle and tingling type pains that are not frequent. I do realize that MRI is not always conclusive and sometimes they need a spinal fluid sample to better evaluate for MS and other neuro-spinal diseases.

Like many people, I feared motor neuron disease as well however, I've searched a great deal on these and they are typically **far more rapidly progressing** than are my symptoms. My muscle fatigability goes back a good 7 years (more likely 10 years) and I've yet to see any hint of atrophy in any muscles (shrinking of them). If mine were an MND (Motor Neuron Disease), it would have to be the slowest progressing on record - even if it was the less-aggressive type. My neurologist suggests "axonal peripheral neuropathy" is what I'm suffering from but he says it is not an absolute. This of course would be a better diagnosis than would something more severe.

Q & A: OPINION FIFTEEN

My Adrenal and Nutritional Lab Evaluations

This article is derived from a forum post, in which I describe lab testing I have received in attempt to diagnose my symptoms of fatigue, muscle weakness and peripheral neuropathy. ---

"They did test my calcium, along with vitamin D level (these two nutrients work together for *bone health*) and it was <u>good range</u>, so they supplemented me with vitamin D, to treat my deficiency of it but no calcium replacement therapy. This-too I believe to be basically a *learn-as-you-practice* thing with my doctor because she was not aware that D-deficiency could cause muscle weakness or nervous system symptoms. She did know that B12 could do this, which I was also found to be low-normal (insufficient) in. I was hoping with the months of treatment for these 3 vitamin deficiencies, that I would have seen more improvement but much of the lingering of symptoms may be related to my *co morbid dysautonomia* (imbalance in my involuntary nervous system) -- which BTW, my past doctors <u>had never heard of</u>, nor has my current one heard of it. I've yet to ask my neurologist but I would suspect that he does know about *disorders of dysautonomia.*

I do love my neurologist however, although he has no clue what level of vitamin E replacement I am supposed to be on, as an ongoing maintenance dose.

This was yet another deficiency I was diagnosed-with, so he is letting me take whatever I think is right (I'm taking 200IU daily) and he'll blood retest it afterward. My vitamin E level was at "0.4" (less than a half point) in a range of 3.0 to 16.0, which can account-for some, if not all of my neurological type problems. Very few doctors know about symptoms or complications of E-deficiency because **it is rare**.

I have longstanding *adrenal fatigue* as well; another issue I've had in regard to doctors not knowing about it and/or not recognizing it as a *real illness*. Mine was found through repeated saliva hormone tests and one 24 hour urinary one but I passed an *ACTH Stimulation Test*, so the low-normal (sometimes flagged low) adrenal cortisol levels were pronounced **"untreatable"**. The ACTH Stimulation test also showed that my pituitary gland responded correctly to the ACTH (Adrenocorticotropic Hormone) with releasing CRH (Corticotropin Releasing Hormone), to stimulate cortisol release from my adrenals. My TSH (another pituitary hormone) responds-well to a lowering or elevation of my thyroid hormones, so this-too was indicative of normal pituitary function. I think they also tested my natural ACTH levels and this too was normal."

NOTE SINCE I MADE THE ABOVE POST: I'm currently treated for D, E and B12 deficiencies and hypothyroidism but I have to self-treat with adrenal supplements when I have flares or chronic episodes of *adrenal fatigue.*

(Note: My neurologist later confirmed that my ongoing maintenance dose of vitamin E should be **from 200 to 250ID daily**, via inquiry he made in regard to it, with his medical colleagues.)

Q & A: OPINION SIXTEEN

My Imbalanced Fear of ALS and Motor Neuron Disease

Like MANY PEOPLE (I know this from forum searches), I feared I might have a Motor Neuron Disease (MND) like ALS (Amyotrophic Lateral Sclerosis) as I mention in the preceding posts and I had some fear about the MS (Multiple Sclerosis) possibility as well. After much online search on the best medical sources, driven by my neurosis in regard to these diseases (a degree of hypochondria) I realized that muscle weakness that goes back as many years as mine does (at least 7 and more likely 10 years) is far too-slow progressing to be a typical MND (I have no muscle atrophy after all that time) but would my symptoms would be more possible for MS or even more possible for a type of polyneuropathy.

My muscle weakness (myopathy) is body-wide (not severe and no foot drop or other severe signs), which is also not typical of an MND. I almost feel bad because I posted on a neurology forum about this concern and the moderating Dr. thought I was saying that my neurologist was concerned about my having an MND.

It was rather I who brought it up to my neuro-doctor and he stated at least twice that my condition is indicative of an **axonal peripheral neuropathy** and not of an MND. I was a little blunt with the forum Dr. but he somehow got the impression that my Dr. was trying to rule-out an MND, which is not the case and I felt I needed to correct that misunderstanding. I was actually asking an opinion on the forum, about my EMG results (Electromyography test) and was asking for comment on that specifically. No big deal, they are extremely busy guys and most donate their time on these medical support type forums.

I also realized there is a kind of fear-mongering (mostly unintentional) directed at people fearing terminal diseases, like those I've described above. I feel people posting on forums, out of fear for what type disease(s) might be affecting them, need replies that are **in-perspective**; otherwise their fears become more deeply imbedded. This is not fair to them. While they do need to know about the more serious, rare types of illnesses, they also need to know how possible these are in comparison to the more common diagnoses, they are more likely to be given.

Q & A: OPINION SEVENTEEN

My Personal Struggle with Myopathy (Muscle Weakness)

The following article is derived from forum posts I made in regard to my personal symptom of myopathy (muscle weakness) and how my thyroid disease and vitamin deficiencies may have played a role in this symptom. ---

Problems with protein and fat metabolism (the use of these designed to be natural energy in the body) can cause vitamin deficiencies and/or muscle problems in the body, like I am experiencing (i.e. weakness and pain symptoms). My blood protein level was checked and was in the upper half of the normal range, indicating that mine is not a protein-metabolism problem. Absorption problems are **a strong possibility** in myopathy cases as well. In other cases they can determine a different cause or find that it's "idiopathic" (no cause determined). I had only a "trace" of protein in my urine lab tests but my regular doctor who had it tested said that trace amounts are commonly found and is only of concern if the amount is significantly high. She also said that if a person has eaten lots of meat or has exercised within 48 hours before a urine test, trace protein and trace red blood cells can be found in the urine. I'm sure that one will still be retested again down the road for me.

Some people also have fat malabsoroption as **a cause** of vitamin deficiencies.

With my being moderately overweight and not having diarrhea problems (a symptom of it), it's <u>not likely</u> to be related to fat metabolism. Still, I asked for a test to detect AMA (anti-mitochonrial antibodies) because these can attack the bile duct in the liver, causing fat malabsorption and deficiencies of fat-soluble vitamins but **I was negative thankfully** (no biliary cirrhosis). For several years, I didn't have insurance and was a self-pay patient, including paying out-of-pocket, fr things like an MRI test I had done in 2007. Fortunately I was able to get BlueCross within months of my developing the peripheral neuropathy (I had only hints of it before that and I didn't recognize it as PN). This can also be a result of my <u>vitamin deficiencies.</u>

Myopathy -- weakness in the body and muscles is commonly <u>a metabolic thing</u> in some cases (as opposed to nutritional deficiencies) and usually there is no treatment for it in many cases but lifestyle changes can help a lot. This is what I have been finding information on recently. Some medical forums I've read information on, have people putting a bit of a scare in others with body weakness, however, there are huge numbers of causes for muscle myopathies other than 'terminal illnesses that can do you in', within a couple or few years (it's still necessary to rule these out however). When you already have conditions in your body like I have, this can already pretty much explain any muscle or body weakness and in many cases people simply have to live with it and **live healthy as possible** to counter-act it.

My peripheral neuropathy symptoms can have my autoimmune thyroid as a cause and my D and E vitamin deficiencies and B12 insufficiency. Replacing these usually helps a lot but long-term deficiencies can leave some permanent nerve damage, especially in regard to E deficiency (mine was at "0.4" in a range of 3.0 to 16.0).

Q & A: OPINION EIGHTEEN

Thorough Evaluation before CFS or Fibromyalgia Diagnosis

I've have always believed that in <u>many cases</u> of patients being given the CFS diagnosis (Chronic Fatigue Syndrome), that there is an underlying health problem that **was not discovered** or even possibly multi-problems. On the other hand, true CFS or CFIDS, I believe to be a disorder of combined neurological, immune dysfunction and endocrine problems and I believe the same to be true of fibromyalgia, which medical sources say has <u>75% crossover similarities</u> with CFS, the main distinction being body pain (FMS), versus fatigue (CFS) as the prominent symptoms.

Some people are not tested for ALL POSSIBLE deficiencies and this can result in a CFS/FMS diagnoses, when the real problem is a deficiency of D, E, B12, B6, Folate, Carnitine, magnesium, potassium, electrolyte imbalances, etc.........

Some CFS patients that are claimed to have been "thoroughly evaluated", were not in-reality tested or examined to the fullest extent for underlying problems.

It is a very intriguing subject but **sad in many ways**. I've done extensive search and research on these sometimes mysterious syndromes and I can understand why the CFS/FMS subject is frustrating even for many doctors. I just hope they don't burn out on research that will bring us who need those "deserved answers someday".

Q & A: OPINION NINETEEN

My Experience with Adult-Onset Asthma

Breathing is regulated by the involuntary nervous system and something we often take for granted. I slowly developed asthma as an adult in my 40s. It is mild-persistent and I only rarely have to use albuterol rescue inhalers. My asthma may have aspects of upper airway resistance involved because when I lay flat on my back - supine, I immediately feel some **tightness in my lungs**. This is however not uncommon with typical asthma, especially in those who also have GERD (Gastro Esophageal Reflux Disease) as I do. It did concern me at first however, because I wanted to make sure there was no heart involvement (enlargement of it) in my asthma, so I had my doctor order me a "BNP" blood test (B-type Natriuretic Peptide), which is **very accurate** for detecting congestive heart and my result was a "4".

I was very happy to see that because elevated readings of 100 can indicate mild heart failure (the lower the result, the better the prognosis). BNP results at from 300 to 600 represent moderate heart enlargement/failure and those at **900 and above**, represent <u>severe cases</u>.

I also had a chest/lung x-ray done (two views) and my lung tissue is healthy, my heart size is normal, with no acute or chronic cardiopulmonary findings.

I've had the acid reflux disease for <u>many years</u> but within months of my adult asthma fully manifesting (I first had it as a child and milder manifestations as an adult), I had several episodes of choking on stomach acid, which made me wheeze and hyperventilate afterward. Medical studies have shown that **75% of asthma patients have GERD** and that GERD is a <u>direct cause</u> of asthma in some people. Vitamin E and D deficiency are believed to also be contributors to asthma as well (possibly <u>direct causes</u>) and I have been diagnosed with both deficiencies (now treated). Still, all-in-all my asthma is mild – and I have so-far never had any severe episodes.

<u>Q & A: OPINION TWENTY</u>

Can the Epstein-Barr Virus Reactivate?

I've found information in regard to EBV (the Epstein-Barr Virus), which has been found to be <u>highly associated</u> with neurological diseases including Multiple Sclerosis.

This includes the fact that in immune-compromised people (having autoimmune disease of any kind or low immune function for any reason) can see the virus **replicate** to higher numbers and in some patients it also **reactivates** - the latter being rare. When I was tested for EBV my result was "218" with normal being <20 (below 20) but at the same time it <u>was not</u> active mononucleosis or reactivated mono, despite being almost 11 times the highest-normal cut-off value. I have Hashimoto's thyroiditis (autoimmune hypothyroidism) and I wanted to see if I had high titers of EBV antibodies in my system, which 'could be' a cause or contributor to my thyroid disease, according to medical research studies.

They have several views in EBV blood testing, of how the virus is present or working the body such as the IGG level etc... and I'm not sure which one points to reactivation, when found to be at high levels in patients being tested. I'm a little limited in knowledge in the area of EBV other than which I've written about it in <u>a few articles</u> but I am convinced **it is a 'direct' cause of autoimmune diseases**, including thyroid ones and there is much medical research to confirm this fact.

It can reactivate rather than just increasing to high levels in a person's system because medical sources say that it can do this, although not commonly. They say that it is more of an occurrence in **"immune-compromised" people** as mentioned previously, meaning insufficient immunity (i.e. aids, Chronic Fatigue Syndrome and if someone has an autoimmune disease or diseases).

Here is a reputable medical quote regarding this:

"Most people, who have infectious mononucleosis, or mono, only get it once. Rarely, however, mononucleosis may recur months or even years later." (Mayo Clinic)

EBV **does reactivate and replicate** in phases in some people who carry it. Some sources say that about <u>80% of people</u> within the general public, carry the virus but that it only reactivates in a small percent and is usually only present in small titers. Some people are carriers and never experienced mono - so the scenarios regarding the virus, range a great deal.

SECTION TWO:
Questions and Answers/Opinions 21 through 40

Q & A: OPINION TWENTY-ONE

Do Low-Normal Cortisol Levels Indicate Adrenal Fatigue?

Derived from a reply I made to someone posting in regard to being found low-normal and clinically-low in adrenal cortisol levels. ---

Cortisol levels are regulated through the adrenal glands via the involuntary nervous system. Some of your cortisol readings (per your post) are not just low-normal but flagged clinically low. This can happen with adrenal fatigue however, to rule out true full-blown adrenal insufficiency, an "ACTH Stimulation Test" would need to be done (a medically supervised test). On the other hand if follow-up retests of your cortisol are done after a couple months or so and normalize by taking adrenal fatigue supplements, this would also rule-out true adrenal dysfunction because you wouldn't be able to get truly dysfunctional adrenals to improve with non-prescription adrenal support but this would require a daily high-dose steroid replacement hormone, as **lifelong treatment**.

I hope I'm not sounding too vague but adrenal support is the type thing that you have to do as a trial to see if it helps because people are different in the fact of what helps them.

Sometimes you have to try more than one type supplement that boosts adrenal function to achieve positive results. Your case is showing to be <u>sub clinical</u>, which is what adrenal fatigue is, rather than "overt" (full blown gland dysfunction) and this is why your doctor is saying there's no treatment for it. Full blown adrenal insufficiency has to be treated with steroid cortisol (corticosteroid) as previously mentioned but treating adrenal fatigue with this drug, **can actually worsen it because it can cause "adrenal suppression".** This is why adrenal gland boosting supplements are the way to go with adrenal fatigue in most cases (some severe cases may actually benefit from cortisol therapy).

There are two supplements that I personally take that have helped me at times I needed them for adrenal fatigue. One is called "Adreset" by Metagenics Company and the other is "Cortico B5 B6" by the same company. If you're in the UK, I'm not sure about the availability of these supplements in your country but you can likely order these online if stores are not carrying them in your area.

Another adrenal support supplement by a reputable company is "Cortitrophin" by Vitamin Research Products Company and they have pharmacists and MDs behind the research and development of their supplements.

There are "adrenal glandular" supplements, usually made from beef/bovine source, also available.

These are supposed to contain **the cells** as well as <u>any hormone</u> found in them that boosts same-glands in humans. I believe they say this occurs because <u>some animal endocrine glands</u> have bio-identical cells to ours.

Those supplements you asked about (per the question in your post) are all usually safe, especially at **the manufacturer's suggested dose** and when <u>monitored</u> for any negative side effects. The only supplement I saw in your list of those you asked about, that can cause hypertension as a side effect is **"licorice root"** but as long as you monitor your BP it should otherwise be a safe supplement. Your physician will likely wean you off of the licorice extract if your cortisol normalizes over time or he may place you on a small ongoing dose after the initial phase of treatment. It probably depends on what your follow up blood retests show.

It's my understanding that "Glycyrrhizin" is a sweat-tasting substance that comes from the licorice plant itself and it is supposed to have <u>anti-viral properties</u> to it, while "Glycyrrhiza" (notice the slight difference in spelling) is from the root of the licorice plant and is the substance that <u>raises cortisol levels</u> in adrenal fatigue sufferers. It's likely safe at the manufacturer's label dose-recommendations but like any herbal, **no two people will react, exactly the same** and so side effects should always be monitored for. One potential side effect of licorice root is hypertension as mentioned previously so blood pressure should be <u>rechecked regularly</u> while you are on the supplement.

In my opinion cortisol in your blood or saliva, should be retested as well with each three month period that the licorice root is being taken. If cortisol levels go too high, **this can cause problems too**.

A physician who can <u>oversee the treatment</u> is always best if that is possible (sometimes it's not).

Q & A: OPINION TWENTY-TWO

Activated, Self-Educated Patients have Better Outcomes

As far as the *"don't research medical issues on your own"* attitude sometimes stated by medical people, both my wife and I were told this in regard to online self-educating but if either of us had not researched about our health disorders, we would be in **serious trouble**. I wish I understood Dr.s motivations for trying to suppress people's need to know about their diseases/disorders and treatments especially those that are potentially <u>life-changing</u>.

I had one of my Dr.s tell me *"you can't believe anything you see on the internet"*, after I had shown him some pages I copied off the Mayo Clinic and Baptist Hospital websites. I had another Dr. actually laugh at me because I researched and listed some things on a sheet to give him at one of my follow up visits. A later visit to him, revealed the very things I showed him earlier on that sheet, that I had co morbid to my thyroid disease and that I requested being tested-for.

I say **"knowledge is power"** but even a dozen 10-minute Dr. Office visits will not give you much to go on, unless you are seeing one of those rare Dr.s that actually does inform you as thoroughly as you need to be. Sorry to unload again regarding this issue but **too many people** are needlessly struggling to get better treatment and this is often not accomplished if they do not get involved actively in their diagnoses and treatments.

Why the need for patient, self-advocacy? – I'll give some examples I witnessed first hand:

My dad-in-law died an early death some years ago, after complaining of moderate symptoms that indicated a heart problem after mowing his lawn. He also complained of a tumor on the back of his head. They scheduled him for heart-valve replacement surgery but found a small mass in his lung during x-rays made before his surgery. They said it was probably just scar tissue and to not worry about it or about the tumor on his head. He died within a few months of the surgery, after **cancer spread aggressively throughout his body**. His kids inquired with his health care providers as to why the cancer wasn't further investigated and rather than answer their questions, the Dr./Hospital simply canceled the bill that was owed for his heart surgery! They knew this was admission by the medical entities involved, of improper care but they didn't pursue it any further because they knew this would not change the fact that he had passed away.

My own mother almost died having a routine colonoscopy procedure. They started the routine test <u>too soon</u> after giving anesthesia and she was screaming; "STOP, I'm still awake"! They gave her more general anesthesia but apparently a dose that was **dangerously high** and her vital signs dropped (respiratory below 60%). A terrified nurse called my dad into her recovery room, to tell him what was happening but she survived thankfully, despite this **potentially fatal error**. The hospital called and apologized only after my mother complained to her regular Doctor about the incident.

My point being, that even medical research groups have stated that patients who are <u>activated and self-educated</u> to a reasonable degree actually receive better care and have better outcomes with health care providers and medical treatments, than do patients who are not self-advocating and partnering with their doctors. <u>Medical errors</u> are a major cause of injury and death in the USA each year but patients can play a part in helping to avoid some of these by offering input in regard to concerns and questions they may have about their symptoms and treatments.

Q & A: OPINION TWENTY-THREE

Brief Description of Adrenal Insufficiency Types

(Derived From a forum post I made in year-2005.) ---

I'm putting this simple and a qualified Dr. could give a better description. --

I believe **"primary"** Addison's disease – adrenal insufficiency (low adrenal hormone levels), would be hypo-functioning of the adrenal glands themselves, whereas, **"secondary"** adrenal insufficiency would be from another cause other than the adrenals, such as a medication a person takes, or dysfunction of another gland that regulates the adrenals, such as the pituitary or hypothalamus gland. So, primary adrenal disease is a problem within the gland itself and a secondary cause affects the adrenals, indirectly.

I think too, that the mid-range for blood cortisol normal value levels (the adrenal stress hormone) is wider than for thyroid testing, so it may very well be easier for them to find a maintenance dose to treat adrenal insufficiency via cortisol/cortical steroid (i.e. prednisone), without lots of adjustments to the hormone replacement, as can happen with hypothyroid treatments. I do believe though that they have patients take **extra dosages** when they are ill with the flu, virus, etc... or if they have a stressful or traumatic event because these things call for increased demand for cortisol. They also usually have you wear a medical I.D. bracelet, in case someone were to find you unconscious, from an accident etc... and they know you could go into an "Addison's Crises" (severe shock from low cortisol) and may need an immediate dose of hormone.

Q & A: OPINION TWENTY-FOUR

Factors Involving Dysautonomia and Orthostatic Hypotension

(Derived from a forum post I made in year-2005.) ---

I thought I would respond to your question about water (hydration). Here's a whole other area I researched back when trying desperately to find answers regarding my own symptom manifestations. Orthostatic Intolerance, is considered a type of "Dysautonomia". This just means a dis-regulation of the involuntary nervous system (autonomic N.S.). There are different types of these dysautonomias, such as one called P.O.T.S. (Postural Orthostatic Tachycardia Syndrome).

ISN'T IT AMAZING, how many different variations of reasons for symptoms a person can have! This is one reason I became somewhat frustrated when researching some of them but I'm beginning to believe most of these so-called "medical disorders" have many of the same root causes. I believe it is dis-regulation of the HPA Axis (Hypothalamus-Pituitary-Adrenal), due to something that gets into the axis and **disrupts it**. This could be autoimmune responses, severe trauma and other serious diseases that place great stress on the adrenals and on the body in-general. Stress is not just a mental or emotional thing, it is also physical and sometimes a combination of all these.

Even positive stress I believe can cause adrenal fatigue (low levels of the stress hormone – cortisol) because our bodies can't tell the difference between good and bad stress. It could be that if our adrenals are weakened, by the stress of something like thyroid disease, it makes them more susceptible to autoimmune attacks and to the non-autoimmune type adrenal insufficiency as well.

Even doctors haven't tied all **these things together** as yet and I certainly don't have anywhere near the knowledge they do but there are so many things that seem to be connected to nervous system and adrenal function. In getting back to my reply Re: "hydration", the dysautonomia information sites I've been to, recommended drinking lots of water, to help with low blood volume (hypovolemia), which can also help with symptoms of an imbalanced involuntary nervous system, especially with sudden drops in blood pressure, which are reported with Mitral Valve Prolapse Syndrome as well (another dysautonomic condition involving a heart murmur).

Q & A: OPINION TWENTY-FIVE

Illnesses that Affect Adrenal Cortisol Levels

(This article is derived from a forum post I made in year-2005.) ---

That is interesting, per your post about being found high in adrenal cortisol level, which can be due to the "alarm phase" of adrenal fatigue (first high cortisol, followed by low levels). To tell you the truth, adrenal insufficiency (eventual low cortisol levels) might be a **better/preferred diagnosis** than Cushing's disease (high cortisol levels) if your case is not that of simple adrenal fatigue because they don't have to do surgery usually to remove a tumor with clinically low cortisol levels; they just give you cortisol hormone replacement medication (the steroid version). It's hard to believe how so many of us go through these yo-yo type revelations about our hormones. First we think they are too high, then too low but its no one's fault, especially when they are doing all the right tests to find the cause for hormone imbalance, as with your case regarding cortisol levels.

I know it is a strange fact but sometimes adrenal insufficiency will result in high blood pressure and sometimes low (low more common). I know this from reading many websites for medical sources on the subject. I think it depends on the "cause". If it is caused by chronic stress, I believe it causes the high blood pressure and weight gain but if it is glandular such as in Addison's disease (dying adrenal glands), weight loss is the result and low blood pressure but HERE AGAIN, this might not be true with each person!

I can't help but to be intrigued by this subject because it seems like a mystery.

I do know that **chronic stress** can cause high cortisol levels that eventually crash, once the adrenals can no longer keep up with the demand, causing adrenal exhaustion. People with anxiety disorders and depression, typically have "high cortisol" levels, whereas, people with Chronic Fatigue Syndrome and Fibromyalgia, have "low cortisol" levels. Many doctors even believe both of these disorders are a result of burnout in the HPA Axis. Other doctors believe these syndromes are variations of thyroid disorder because CFS and FM are more common in thyroid patients than in any other group of people being studied.

I didn't mean to rattle on, but this low adrenal thing has some amazing connections to it. Some websites state that about **10% of hypothyroid patients** have a degree of co-existing adrenal insufficiency. Another one stated that 25% (1 in 4) Hashimoto's thyroiditis patients (autoimmune hypothyroidism) often develop co-existing conditions, adrenal insufficiency being in that list of possibilities. I hope doctors start tying some of this together better soon for all of us!

I will be VERY interested to know what your "adrenal antibodies" reading is, when results come back. This is the very test I am thinking about getting done myself!

(NOTE: I actually did have this test done months following this post and I was negative for autoimmune adrenal disease.)

<u>Q & A: OPINION TWENTY-SIX</u>

Degrees of Cortisol Deficiency Associated with Health Disorders

Chronic Fatigue Syndrome and Fibromyalgia are examples of two different types of illnesses that have <u>varied degrees</u> of adrenal insufficiencies associated with them and they are also often tied somehow into thyroid function. An endocrine gland "axis" I hear some of the medical sources refer-to, is the "Thyroid-Adrenal Axis". Some also refer to the HPA Axis (Hypothalamus-Pituitary-Adrenal).

Here's a couple more interesting facts in that area; The National Institutes of Health (Allergies & Infectious Diseases Dept), did a study on CFS (Chronic Fatigue Syndrome) in 1996 and they state in their Embargoed Release, that "CFS Patients had slightly lower levels of circulating cortisol...than healthy individuals". They also said; "Doctors have long known that <u>even subtle deficiencies</u> in cortisol can be associated with lethargy and fatigue". They also said; "...low cortisol levels in the CFS patients MIGHT be due to deficiencies in cortitropin-releasing-hormone (CRH), a brain chemical that helps regulate cortisol secretion." (Note: CRH is not the same as the ACTH blood level and they don't have a test for measuring it).

Another department of the National Institutes of Health - "NIAMS" (Arthritis, Musculoskeletal and Skin Diseases Dept.), found the same research results with Fibromyalgia.

They stated that "...low levels of the hormone cortisol may be associated with fibromyalgia." They also said that "People whose bodies make inadequate amounts of cortisol experience the same symptoms as people with fibromyalgia." What I am leaning toward in my understanding of these research studies, is that some people with CFS and FM type symptoms may have a sub-clinical form of adrenal insufficiency associated with them.

Did you know that President John F. Kennedy, developed adrenal insufficiency after being shot down, as a fighter pilot in WWII? He was afterward placed on replacement adrenal hormone therapy from that point forward, until his death in 1963. Some people can experience a severe stressor that causes adrenal insufficiency or chronic, prolonged stressors. Post Traumatic stress Disorder (PTSD) which is considered to be an "anxiety condition" has also been found to present with low cortisol levels that contribute to its symptoms. Many people with CFS and FM, report that they had a viral-illness that seemed to **trigger it**, similar to a severe allergic reaction or a flu type illness. My belief is that thyroid disease (autoimmune), both Graves' disease and Hashimoto's thyroiditis possibly triggers this same type of adrenal problem in some patients who develop them.

Q & A: OPINION TWENTY-SEVEN

A Few Fast Facts for Anxiety Sufferers

As terrible as anxiety feels, it is **neither harmful nor dangerous**. Using that sentence as a search, you'll see multiple sites confirming this fact. Anxiety is a natural emotion, created to help us flee from danger or to perform more powerfully for an important task (fight or flight response). With "anxiety disorder" this mechanism happens at the wrong times, such as at the grocery store check out stand, in a crowd of people etc... Anxiety and depression commonly co-exist, in fact more people with anxiety disorders have depression than don't. Anxiety will not make you go crazy, no matter how often you experience it and it will not cause you physical damage, unless you already have serious underlying health problems (still a low possibility). It heightens bodily functions the same as exercise does. Anxiety is not stress - it is a manifestation of stress and is the body's way of trying to shed-off stressful things by allowing the body to react to them.

Sometimes with strong anxiety emotions, people experience "depersonalization and/or derealization", in which one feels unreal or everything around them feels unreal (unreality symptoms). This is not a sign of insanity; it is common with anxiety and depression. Anxiety will not progress to schizophrenia or insanity because it is "neurosis" and not "psychosis" which are **two completely different things**.

People with "psychosis" may have no anxiety or depression at all. Psychosis is defined by delusions and hallucinations. Anxiety suffers can have mild hallucination-type experiences but this is the minds way of trying to locate a perceived danger and it is still not the same as true psychosis. These facts comforted me greatly at times of severe anxiety I experienced with the onset of Hashimoto's thyroiditis in year 2003, that first manifested with severe anxiety and panic symptoms (Hashitoxicosis). I hope it helps you out there with anxiety struggles, who may read this as well.

Q & A: OPINION TWENTY-EIGHT

Saliva Duct Stones Associated with Autoimmune Diseases

My forum post Re: "Saliva Duct Stones Associated with Autoimmune Diseases".---

Saliva production is yet another bodily function that is regulated by the involuntary nervous system. I had a saliva duct stone when I was about 7 years of age that a doctor removed in his office. Again I had one when I was about age-35 and I hate to admit it but I removed that one it myself (I should have sought professional medical treatment).

It seems to me that I've read on some medical sources, that Sjogren's Syndrome (an autoimmune disease of bodily dryness) does cause saliva-duct stones in **some people**.

In fact I believe I read this in Mary Shomon's book titles: "Living Well with Autoimmune Disease", which I highly recommend. She details how that Sjogren's is also an autoimmune disease in which antibodies attack mucous membranes, causing severe dry mouth, eyes and lack of adequate moisture anywhere else in the body. I have never had Sjogren's, so I don't know what my duct stones were caused by. I do know it caused me **significant pain** under my tongue and in my throat because saliva builds up in the glands that produce it and has no where else to go. Eating was sometimes painful as well, when I had these duct stones. People with autoimmune thyroid diseases, are at higher risk for developing Sjogren's and other autoimmune disorders, than is the healthy public.

Q & A: OPINION TWENTY-NINE

Some Quick Facts about Asthma

While we can consciously change our breathing patterns, it is also an involuntary bodily function, regulated by the nervous system (i.e. while we sleep). There is no cure for asthma, which can negatively affect our flow of breathing but it is usually a lifelong disease. Some asthma patients do however see the condition vary in severity, with months at a time not manifesting with flares or significant symptoms. Some asthmatics experience symptoms more-so in cold months of the year or in those when allergens are at their highest (i.e. mold and pollen).

Pets and household chemicals can also trigger asthma flares. Research studies have shown that up to **75%** of people with asthma have acid reflux as well and they know for a fact that it can be a trigger for it. A trigger meaning it brings it to the surface and aggravates it but **doesn't necessarily cause it.**

Other studies cite GERD as a suspected - direct cause of asthma. I personally saw my adult-onset asthma manifest after several months of worsening acid reflux in which on several occasions I awoke at night choking on stomach acid which burned my throat and caused my lungs to tighten and wheeze. This was occurring despite my taking Prolosec, the prescription-strength over-the-counter acid blocker drug. I feel I was having mild asthma for years previous, I just didn't recognize it as such. Asthma can also worsen bronchial infections from colds or allergy flares.

A qualified Dr. can rule-out other less common causes of asthma with chest x-rays and other tests. These will also rule out heart-involvement which is rare, especially if you haven't experienced a heart attack or heart valve problems and if you are not elderly. If you are a smoker, chronic bronchitis can be present as well and can co-exist with asthma. To repeat, there's no cure for asthma but it can be well-controlled with treatment. Lung infections in asthmatic patients will resolve completely over time with treatment but this usually means they are susceptible to them with colds and flu (bronchitis).

I'm a layperson and not a medical professional but these comments come from a great deal of search on reputable medical research sources.

Q & A: OPINION THIRTY

Can Acid Reflux Disease Trigger Development of Asthma?

My response that follows below was to someone asking about the connection of their GERD to asthma symptoms, which they developed after contracting a flu virus. ---

(Note: Stomach acid production and the function of the esophagus are moderated by the involuntary nervous system.)

This is layperson, non-med pro opinion of course but one thing that comes to mind is that your years of GERD (as described in your post) may have started some inflammation in your lungs but it had not yet manifested as asthma. The flu virus may have been a trigger that brought the asthma to the surface that was in a sense **dormant**. I know that when asthma manifested in me about a year ago, I could remember times past that I had mild indications of it. I in fact remember one particular asthma flare that occurred several years ago and I wondered at that time if an allergen triggered a solitary flare. I now believe the asthma was there for quite some time, it just took a while for it to **fully reveal itself**. I believe adult asthma can have a slow onset.

Severe cases of GERD should be evaluated by a Gastroenterologist.

Gastroenterologists specialize in the diagnosis and treatment of health disorders affecting the large and small intestines and esophageal disorders (affecting the esophagus). These would be conditions such as Irritable Bowel Syndrome, Crohn's disease, Ulcers, Gastro esophageal Reflux Disease (acid reflux), parasites, colon cancer (malignancy may also require an Oncologist) and other disorders of the digestive system.

Gastroenterology is the practice these doctors specialize-in by providing definitive diagnoses through tests such as upper and lowers G.I.s (Barium x-rays), colonoscopies and blood lab testing. Once they have diagnosed conditions present in patients, they can then give them the **appropriate treatments**, which may include drug therapies, specialized diets and/or surgeries to control symptoms or to resolve the conditions.

Q & A: OPINION THIRTY-ONE

Are There Effective Natural Anxiety Treatments?

Yes, there are natural supplements, including some herbals that are reported to be helpful to some anxiety patients by calming the nervous system. I mention some of these in other anxiety-subject articles. I do however believe that a person should **approve any supplement** through their doctor.

The U.S. National Institutes of Health, lists natural supplements on one of their sites, explaining their uses and what they have learned about them through their research. It is a reputable source for the evaluation of natural supplements in my opinion. Here are two anxiety herbals they give information on and you can find others using their alphabetized categories at the top of these pages.

(MedLine Plus – Drugs and Supplements "Valerian"), Quote: *"Several studies of valerian have reported benefits in reducing non-specific anxiety symptoms."*

(MedLine Plus – Drugs and Supplements "Kava"), Quote: *"Human studies have found at least moderate benefit of kava in the treatment of anxiety, and early evidence suggests that kava may be as effective as benzodiazepine drugs such as diazepam (Valium®)."*

Q & A: OPINION THIRTY-TWO

Can Autoimmune Thyroiditis cause Neuropathy?

Neurological symptoms can occur with thyroid autoimmunity and is a fact confirmed by a condition called "Hashimoto's Encephalopathy" which although rare, causes severe neurological symptoms. In Graves' disease, patients commonly experience optic neuropathy of the eyes. It would seem obvious that neuro-symptoms to lesser degrees can also occur.

The MRI you had was valuable in ruling out neurological diseases and as far as treatments go, published medical research has shown that **selenium supplementation** can help reduce thyroid antibodies, so one should discuss this mineral for becoming part of their treatment regimen, with their treating doctor.

Otherwise, patients with severely elevated antibodies are sometimes treated with corticosteroid anti-inflammatory drugs (cortical steroids) such as the brand called "Prednisone", as short-term therapy. Some <u>severe cases</u> of neurological symptoms and neuropathies, are treated with drugs designed to address them, such a "Neurontin". In some cases antidepressants are used, such as the brand "Cymbalta". Of course all of these are <u>prescription treatments</u> and must be administered by a medical doctor if he feels any of them would be a benefit to a thyroid patient with neuropathy symptoms.

<u>Q & A: OPINION THIRTY-THREE</u>

About Bipolar Depressive Disorder

Medical research is ongoing to find definitive causes for Bipolar Disorder which certainly involves brain and nervous system involvement. Bipolar disorder is a **mental disorder** that manifests just as the name implies - "bi" meaning <u>two poles</u>. The poles are opposite in that a bipolar person becomes **extremely depressed** during their mood disorder episodes but they become highly elated during their **manic episodes**.

For most bipolar people, they experience these alternating phases/poles for days at a time but some experienced a more rapid cycling of these or "mixed episodes".

So, if you experience both severe (major) depression and times of opposite elation, this could mean bipolar but a mental health evaluation can determine it with more certainty. Just to add - the elation from manic episodes can make a person want to go on shopping sprees or to work on creative projects for days at a time and they may find it difficult to sleep because of the "high feeling". They may also have **delusions** at these times.

Bipolar, unlike typical emotional disorders that are in the "neurosis" category (i.e. anxiety disorders and major depression) in some cases can actually be considered a condition of intermittent psychosis (times of delusions or hallucinations). This means it is a lifelong mental disorder likely caused by subtle brain abnormalities, which means psychotropic drug treatment is **life-long**.

Some bipolar cases are more severe than others and some patients are treated with only an antidepressant like an SSRI (Selective Serotonin Reuptake Inhibitor) while others may also need an anti-psychotic drug. With proper, ongoing treatment, bipolar patients can lead normal, productive lives.

<u>Q & A: OPINION THIRTY-FOUR</u>

A Brief Look at Non-Alcoholic Fatty Liver

(NOTE: The liver is an involuntary nervous system regulated organ.)

A common follow up test ordered for people suspected of having <u>fatty liver disease</u> is one called "liver ultrasound" and this can confirm fatty liver when the dark redish-colored organ has a slick appearance to it, since healthy livers have a dull appearance. It can also detect whether any tumors or lesions appear on it. This is actually more of a precaution because NAFLD (non-alcoholic fatty liver disease) is very common and the majority of cases <u>do not</u> progress to physically harmful or life-threatening conditions. A liver biopsy, in which they extract a small tissue sample via a fine needle, is usually not ordered unless **lesions or spots are found** via ultrasound.

If your readings on two commonly ordered liver enzyme blood tests called the "ALT" and "AST", are not elevated more than a few points above the normal range, a doctor might not even deem an ultrasound necessary because that's not twice or three times the highest normal value (depending on normal range) and is not usually considered significant if there **is not a high elevation** or accompanying symptoms such as pain on the right side of the abdomen.

Another reason to follow up with a doctor if one does experience pain they suspect to be caused by the liver is due to the possibility of the pancreas or gallbladder being involved but. In most cases it involves the liver-only, which is located in the front-shank area, on the right side. Cases of advanced fatty liver, both alcoholic and non-alcoholic types can cause swelling and may do so after eating fatty foods or those that are spicy or that contain things the body recognizes as **toxins**.

Fatty liver in most cases is benign but in rare cases can progress to "fatty liver hepatitis", also called "NASH" (Non-Alcoholic Fatty Liver Steto-hepatitis). While pain in this area could be something as simple as Irritable Bowel Syndrome, a visit to a qualified doctor can give one peace on mind, as he rules out serious causes.

Q & A: OPINION THIRTY-FIVE

Can Anxiety Disorders be Medically Caused?

There are a number of medical causes for anxiety, including neurotransmitter imbalances and your doctor can evaluate you for these. Some of these causes would also include sex hormone imbalances, thyroid disorders, blood glucose imbalances and a common heart murmur called "Mitral Valve Prolapse", which often involves a nervous system imbalance called "dysautonomia".

While psychotropic drugs like antidepressants and anti-anxiety medications can be effective in treating anxiety disorders, if there is an underlying medical condition contributing-to or directly causing your anxiety symptoms, diagnosing and treating it can go further than any other treatment in resolving it.

If other causes are ruled-out, one can discuss with their doctor, a trial of a medication directed a relieving anxiety symptoms or psychiatric and self-help therapies that can help to accomplish this. Many anxiety patients benefit from a combination of both and in some cases can wean-off slowly from medication, once other therapies have gained them ample coping skills. SSRI antidepressants (drugs that regulate neurotransmitters in the brain) for example **do not benefit everyone** who is give a trial of them and some are switched to other types, such as non-addictive, long term anti-anxiety medications, one called BuSpar (or generic-Busperone), being in that category.

Q & A: OPINION THIRTY-SIX

Can Hypoglycemia Mimic a Psychiatric Disorder?

Glucose (blood sugar) is regulated in the body through **the pancreas** (endocrine gland that produces insulin) via the involuntary nervous system. While "hypoglycemia" (a sudden drop in blood glucose levels) doesn't mimic bipolar to a large degree, a person can experience "highs and lows" from fluctuations in glucose levels.

When glucose goes low for example, the brain is starved of this **very essential element** for its proper functioning and can cause the person having the hypoglycemic episode to act strangely and present with spells of <u>bizarre behaviors</u>. Severe hypoglycemia can actually cause a person to **hallucinate** and to experience short term memory loss.

People with wide swings in glucose have also been known to <u>pass out</u> and if not treated, they can also risk <u>diabetic coma</u>. Hypoglycemia also causes adrenaline surges, which is the body's way of trying to compensate for low glucose, which can produce obvious **anxiety symptoms**. Adversely, hyperglycemic episodes (too much glucose in the blood) can make a person feel sleepy - both being the opposite of what you would think should happen. These factors might cause the one observing them to think they are experiencing **a mental or emotional disorder**.

Q & A: OPINION THIRTY-SEVEN

A Brief Look at Schizophrenia

Schizophrenia is an illness affecting the mind and emotions that causes episodes of delusions, hallucinations and fragmented thinking or detached thoughts.

This form of mental illness <u>is treatable</u> and treatment can actually reduce symptoms of psychosis to a degree that patients can live relatively normal lives.

It is very important however, that treatment is adhered-to **exactly as scheduled** because missed doses of drug therapies can hinder the effects of it.

There are certain diseases that can be mistaken for schizophrenia, including thyroid disorders, especially the ones called "Hashimoto's Encephalopathy" (an acute neurological disease) and "Thyroid Storm". The same is true of severe **nutritional deficiencies** that can cause psychosis until diagnosed and treated. Severe Vitamin D deficiency for example has been identified as a cause of schizophrenia in medical research studies and correction of it via Vitamin D replacement therapy can resolve it.

In these type cases, treating underlying medical disorders can cure the mental illness but when schizophrenia does not have an underlying cause but is "idiopathic" (its own disorder - no secondary cause), it is lifelong and requires ongoing treatment.

Q & A: OPINION THIRTY-EIGHT

Potential Symptoms of Gastro Esophageal Reflux Disease

Acid Reflux Disease is also called "GERD" (Gastro Esophageal Reflux Disease) and is a condition in which stomach acid and sometimes undigested foods **move upward** from the stomach, into the esophagus. This causes acid indigestion and heartburn, especially in the supine position (lying down flat).

The symptoms can include heart burn, difficulty swallowing, a bad taste in the mouth, mild chest pain, sore throat, mild laryngitis and episodes of waking at night due to **choking and breathing difficulties**.

The breathing problems related to GERD are due to small amounts of acid and food particles entering into the lungs from the windpipe. The esophageal valve in the throat that closes off when eating, to prevent food from entering the windpipe, is called "the sphincter" but with GERD, this valve begins to relax and not seal-off properly, causing acid to enter the lungs. This can eventually cause asthma symptoms and medical research studies have shown that **approximately 75%** of asthma patients also suffer from GERD. Some studies state that GERD is a direct cause of respiratory problems while others state that it is an aggravating factor for them.

The severity of GERD can be determined via a "barium swallow" test and/or an endoscope/bronchoscope procedure if breathing difficulties have resulted. If GERD has been severe, a condition will need to be ruled out via these tests called "Barrett's Esophagus" - a pre-cancerous condition that can develop as damage occurs to the esophagus.

Q & A: OPINION THIRTY-NINE

Why is my Asthma Aggravated by Laying Flat?

I had asthma as a child and then afterward, not for many years and then again as a middle-aged adult. I have also had GERD (acid reflux), for <u>many years</u> which I believe to have either **caused or aggravated** my asthma (medical research strongly confirms the connection). What seriously concerned me, until I had tests done by my doctor to <u>rule out a serious problem</u>, was a worsening of my asthma immediately upon lying flat on my back ("orthopnea").

I had my doctor order chest x-ray and a "BNP" blood test (B-type natriuretic peptide) to <u>rule out</u> **the possibility** of any degree of <u>heart failure</u> (cardiac asthma) and my tests <u>were negative</u> for any heart involvement in my asthma. I find many medical sources saying GERD is highly associated with asthma and that GERD can cause orthopnea but little on sources in regard to asthma itself (the common garden variety) causing more breathing difficulty when laying flat on ones back. My suspicion is that it's a <u>fairly common</u> thing with asthma and other lung diseases/disorders.

I also feel anxiety feelings at times that come from anticipating the chest tightness and constriction of the bronchial tubes which can actually **trigger more asthma** when one lays flat (at least for those of us with co morbid anxiety).

My asthma returned in my forties (I'm now in my 50s) and as far as **propping up on pillows**, I too find relief doing that. I can more comfortably lay on my sides or stomach but can still experience a degree of chest tightness in these positions if my asthma is flaring (more-so on my back) but my albuterol inhaler relieves it a great deal, in preparing for a night's sleep.

Additionally, some medical sources state that the **same nerve endings** affect both the esophagus and lungs and that irritated nerves may send a signal to the lungs to close more, when one takes the supine position as a protection mechanism, to prevent damage to them from any acid that seeps into the windpipe. The lungs in-essence develop learned behaviors after repeated exposure to small amounts of stomach acid as kind of a **self-preservation reaction**.

Q & A: OPINION FORTY

What Causes Mildly Elevated Liver Enzymes?

If the ALT and/or AST are only mildly elevated, the most common cause is "non-alcoholic fatty liver", which affects all ages, **including young children** and is commonly associated with obesity. This condition is not actually one of liver damage but of very mild inflammation and very small amounts of cell death in the organ due to fatty infiltration.

If they are highly elevated - at least double the highest high-normal cut off value, this can indicate liver disease, such as one of the many types of hepatitis, alcoholism, certain illegal and prescription drug usages and anything else that causes **damage to the organ.** Fatty liver can also progress to a type of hepatitis, referred to as NASH (Non-Alcoholic Fatty Liver Steato-Hepatitis) but this is rare compared to typical fatty liver.

The normal value range for "Direct bilirubin" is appoximately: "0 to 0.3 mg/dL" and for "Total bilirubin", it is: "0.3 to 1.9 mg/dL" and an elevation above normal values of theses tests **can also indicate liver disease** or bile duct blockage which most commonly occurs when one has gall stones.

The normal range value range for "Alkaline Phosphate" is "44 to 147 IU/L" and when it elevates above normal values, this too can also mean bile duct obstruction from **gall stones**.

Of course these two blood levels can elevate for other reasons as well, such as liver disease, bone problems, anemia and cancer but gall stones are by far the most common reason for elevations in them.

SECTION THREE:
Questions and Answers/Opinions 41 through 60

Q & A: OPINION FORTY-ONE

How Do You Support a Person with Bipolar Disorder?

Bipolar patients need total support that they can sense and feel from you and being available to listen when they need to talk and offering words of encouragement as often as necessary, is important. Also giving them space to be alone when they legitimately need private time to themselves and there is **no danger** that they will harm their self. Reassuring them that their drug therapy is essential to their ongoing health and that it is helping them to retain a better quality-of-life is important.

Complimenting them, on their accomplishments and encouraging them to continue achieving personal goals as they are able to do so **is also part of this**. Reminding them that they are not "insane" or "crazy" but that they have a **mental illness** which does not take away from their inward character or intelligence can be beneficial. Letting them know often that you love them if your relationship allows, can also be supportive.

Bipolar is possibly something one has at birth and is a lifelong disorder. Some medical research has shown that the brains of bipolar patients reveal differences from that of the healthy general public.

But **no definitive conclusions** have been made as yet in regard to brain differences. Despite it being a lifelong disorder, it may not manifest in some people until adult years. Most cases have become evident by the time a person reaches their early twenties.

Q & A: OPINION FORTY-TWO

Can Having Low Blood Pressure be Unhealthy?

(Note: blood pressure is regulated by the INS and is highly influenced by the "sympathetic branch".)

Low blood pressure (hypotension) is often idiopathic - meaning it has **no actual cause** that can be determined. Not being well-hydrated can cause low blood volume (hypovolemia) and resulting hypotension (low blood pressure). Low blood sodium levels (hyponatremia) can cause hypotension as well. Certain types of dysfunction of the involuntary nervous system, also referred-to as "dysautonomia" can cause low blood pressure as well and people with a common heart murmur called "Mitral Valve Prolapse" often have a type of dysautonomia that occurs with it.

Low blood pressure begins at "90 over 60" and below. Anything above that is not typically dangerous, such as levels of "100 over 65", etc... Very low blood pressure can place a person at risk for stroke, due to **lack of blood** reaching the brain, otherwise moderately low blood pressure is much healthier than high blood pressure – "hypertension".

Q & A: OPINION FORTY-THREE

Is Daily Coffee Drinking Unhealthy for the Nervous System?

Coffee consumed in moderation is not unhealthy unless you have a pre-existing condition that causes it to have adverse reactions in your body. If you have acid reflux disease (GERD) for example, coffee that may be consumed close to bedtime can cause heartburn symptoms to **due it being acidic**.

If a person has a weak heart, such as is seen with enlargement of it or congestive heart failure, coffee consumption might be recommended against, due to its stimulating effect on the body and nervous system (i.e. sympathetic branch that regulates adrenaline production and release.) which might place extra stress on an already **weak heart muscle**. Otherwise, in healthy people, coffee should not have a negative effect on the heart, unless consumed in extremely large quantities.

GERD can be well-controlled in most cases, using acid blocking drugs, also referred to as "proton pump inhibitors" and "H2 blockers". Avoiding spicy foods and caffeine can also help, as can elevating the head of your bed by about six inches. This can be done by placing bricks or books under the headboard legs.

Q & A: OPINION FORTY-FOUR

How Can one Manage Chronic Fatigue and Stress?

See your doctor for a complete physical and ask for **blood testing** of your blood counts (CBC) to see if there might be a type of anemia present, an averaged glucose level (HB-A1C) to see if diabetes might be present, a thyroid panel to see if you might have hypothyroidism (under active) and the major vitamin levels (B12, D and E) to see if you have nutritional deficiencies. If nothing is revealed in these, you might need a follow up blood panel to test your sex hormone levels and the type that detect inflammation and/or tissue damage in the body (i.e. The ESR, ANA, CK, RA Factor, liver, heart and kidney function blood tests).

If it is found that you're healthy and not in need of treatment for a health disorder, you should do everything you can to **improve your diet**, eating less to no junk foods and adding more fruits, vegetable, nuts and grains and **eliminating stimulants** like caffeine, alcohol and refined sugars. Taking good multivitamin and safe supplements, containing things that help **increase energy in the body** can help. Also get plenty of rest and adequate sleep (at least 8-hours per night - uninterrupted) and exercise regularly by at least getting 20 minute walks three times a week or by jogging, biking or hiking. The fresh air and taking in some nature and beauty will also serve to **reduce excess stress**. Hobbies, art-pursuits and leisure activities can help in this area as well.

Q & A: OPINION FORTY-FIVE

Excessive Thirst and Grandparents with Diabetes and Lupus

Can this combination of factors increase the risk for these diseases in a third generation grandson (a question asked on behalf of the person's son)?

(Note: glucose regulation in the body is accomplished via the INS, which regulates the endocrine system, including pancreatic activity.)

Yes, intense thirst itself can point to diabetes (but is not a "cause" of it), however with his grandparents having the adult onset type this would not necessarily place him at higher risk. While endocrine diseases do run in families, type I diabetes which has an autoimmune aspect to it would be more of an inherited disorder.

The thirst itself could be **simple dehydration** and he hasn't been taking time through the day to drink enough water because he is too busy playing and is playing catch-up at the dinner table. Cravings for sugar can of course be caused by hypoglycemia or diabetes and medical sources now recognize that hypoglycemia can occur without the presence of diabetes. One name for it is "reactive hypoglycemia" and it can actually be caused by eating too much refined sugar in the first place (added sugars, not occurring naturally in foods or beverages). Once one indulges in sugar, for energy, the body begins to crave it because **it raises serotonin levels** in the brain.

A person usually indulges in refined refined sugars due to stress or simply because they crave a "carbohydrate high" but they have to **unlearn this behavior** in order to overcome the craving and this can cause a degree of withdrawal.

These may be reasons he is craving hydration and sugar but to be on the safe side, I would get his fasting blood glucose level tested as a precaution (a morning level,before any food is consumed).

Lupus, which you also asked about, is a **multi-organ disease** or systemic (body wide) so that the immune system is attacking multiple areas of normal tissue, such as endocrine glands (hormone-producing). The pancreas is an endocrine gland that supplies the hormone insulin, for converting sugar (glucose) into energy. Lots of Lupus patients are also diabetic but being diabetic does not necessarily point to developing Lupus.

Q & A: OPINION FORTY-SIX

Differences between Bipolar Disorder Types I and II

Both conditions present with **severe episodes of depression**, also referred-to as clinical or major depression and both also present with the opposite pole of emotion, being that of **"mania"**, which are episodes of elation that alternate with the depression. Bipolar II is differentiated due to its less pronounced manic episodes.

They refer to these less severe mania symptoms as "hypomania" because it falls short of causing the severity of mania that those with "bipolar I" have. People with "bipolar II" are also <u>less-prone</u> to experience delusions and/or hallucinations (psychotic episodes).

Bipolar in-general would not simply be depressed mood but would be severely depressed mood, alternating with episodes of an exaggerated mood of elation. Bipolar patients have <u>very unstable moods</u> that go very low and then very high and during the high or "manic" episodes, they may feel greater and mightier than others around them (delusional). The depressed moods can be so severe, as to land a bipolar person in bed for days or weeks at a time and the manic episodes can keep them from sleeping for periods that long as well. The goal of treatment is to get the moods on **a more even level** so that the peaks and valleys are no longer occurring.

<u>Q & A: OPINION FORTY-SEVEN</u>

Can Bipolar Disorder be Misdiagnosed?

If you have extremely depressed episodes, followed by extremely elated episodes (manic/mania), this can point strongly toward bipolar disorder. If you instead have anxiety symptoms that alternate with depression, <u>this would not be bipolar</u> because anxiety is a <u>fear or worry emotion</u> and **not one of elation**.

So, if you cycle between great sadness and an exaggerated happiness that is not triggered by events going on in your life, you may indeed have bipolar disorder, that would be recognized by a mental health professional.

Some people who exhibit episodes of extreme depression, with alternating episodes of anxiety that causes others around them to mis-perceive their nervous energy as "mania", may believe that person is experiencing bipolar, when **they are not**. Doctors have been known to misdiagnose sufferers of combined anxiety and depression, due this very type of **mistaken observation**.

There are some theories that drug and/or alcohol abuse can actually cause bipolar disorder in susceptible people. It is otherwise a brain abnormality that one is born-with but that may not manifest until young adulthood. When I say "born with" this can actually mean that the abnormal components in the brain are **present at birth** but it might not be developed enough to cause the mood swings until early childhood, adolescence or the early adult years.

Q & A: OPINION FORTY-EIGHT

What causes Blood Spots in Sputum (Coughed-up Phlegm from the Mouth)?

It might be a benign lung lesion or tumor that will heal itself over time or it could be a malignant one (cancerous). A severe longstanding cold or allergy that turns into bronchitis can cause mild lung hemorrhage.

This is however, more common with **pneumonia**. If you have one of these lung illnesses, you would likely also run a high fever.

Chronic bronchitis and COPD are breathing diseases that can cause blood spots in the phlegm (sputum) in some people who suffer with them, as can **tuberculosis**. Regardless it is definitely something that should be looked-into by a qualified doctor.

Also: allergens are the most common perpetrators of causing asthma attacks. The only thing I would add to the list of asthma triggers, is strong emotional expressions such as stress, anxiety and even laughter according to some medical sources. Some of them actually refer to asthma triggered by anxiety, as "anxiety induced asthma".

Q & A: OPINION FORTY-NINE

Can Chiari Malformation affect Lifespan Expectancy?

Chiari Malformation, like other diseases or syndromes that affect a person neurologically will not necessarily shorten one's lifespan. It actually depends on whether or not **serious complications develop** such as paralysis, shifting of spinal fluid in the body or breathing problems (i.e. sleep apnea). Usually, with monitoring by a doctor and treatment for any complications that may develop, a person can live a full lifespan.

In spite of this fact, the ongoing symptoms can at times affect a person's quality-of-life and can be disrupting when flares of symptoms occur. This is why a qualified doctor is important in its <u>treatment</u>.

With type II Chiari Malformation affecting newborns, their chances of survival are much lower due to the condition affecting their <u>undeveloped organs</u> **more severely**.

<u>Q & A: OPINION FIFTY</u>

Underarm Pain that Radiates to the Elbow

Pain in the armpit that radiates toward the elbow, can be caused by a pinched nerve, arthritis in the shoulder or a tumor in the breast or surrounding area, **this presses on a nerve**, causing what is referred to as "referred pain" (felt in others areas in addition to the area it originates from). If might also be caused by a muscle that is tensing (tonus/hypertonus) and the striation is one that runs from the armpit to the elbow, such as a bicep. It's also possible that the pain is referred from the forearm (lateral antebrachial cutaneous nerve) rather than the armpit, since nerves can make it difficult at times to determine the **origin of pain**.

A qualified doctor can help to zero-in on the source of the pain through physical examination and/or medical lab testing.

There are also <u>neurological diseases</u> that are autoimmune in nature as well, that cause the "myelin sheath" covering nerves to deteriorate over time, causing nerve damage. Treatment for these types can **improve symptoms** and even reverse some or all of the damage.

Diabetic neuropathies can occur if you have diabetes but this type will usually start in the feet, rather than in one arm. Yours does sound like **a pinched spinal nerve**, based on medical descriptions I have seen but <u>a neurologist</u> could zero-in on it for you, in determining whatever/wherever the problem may be originating from.

<u>Q & A: OPINION FIFTY-ONE</u>

What Does Chest and Arm Pain with Difficulty Breathing Indicate?

I would be very concerned if I experienced <u>that set of symptoms together</u> because that could indicate a **heart attack**. I would handle it by going to a hospital ER because if it is heart-related, they can administer treatment, to <u>prevent further heart damage</u> and possibly **save a person's life**.

On the other hand, those symptoms can also indicate <u>something benign</u>, such as a panic attack. Unless a person knows this, following an initial attack, they would not know that it wasn't their heart, so should seek emergency care **immediately**.

If chronic anxiety is diagnosed, they could then simply deal with further attacks with anti-anxiety medication and/or anxiety coping methods, such as relaxation techniques, slowed deep breathing from the diaphragm, and diversion methods (things that draw attention away from anxiety symptoms).

Q & A: OPINION FIFTY-TWO

Teen Drug Experimentation and "Bad Trips"

(Note: Illegal or irresponsible drug use can result in permanent damage to the nervous system and some medical sources believe that 'some' cases of conditions such as Bipolar Disorder can be directly linked to brain abnormalities resulting from use of some types of these drugs and from chronic alcohol abuse. This should not be misunderstood to mean that all bipolar patients are substance abusers because **this is not the case**.)

When I was a teen in the 1970s, my friends and I were huffing CO_2 from a balloon after filling it with the gas. I don't even remember how we got it but I was breathing in a lot of it at one point and I had what I can only describe as **a very bad trip**. It was as if I was engulfed in a thick, dark-green fog and I heard this loud, echoing banging sound, kind of like a heavy metal door being slammed shut repeatedly. All I could do was wrap my arms around my head while lying on the floor, until these effects went away but **it scared me out of my wits** (I'm glad it did!).

I was afraid I was going to be stuck permanently in this horrible bad trip, which would have definitely been a living hell, had I experienced and survived an <u>ongoing episode</u> of it. My friends thought I was kidding around with the writhing on the floor episode but I wasn't and it terrified me!

I did also freak out on pot once, smoking it with my oldest brother when I was in my early teens. I had the sensation that my left foot was tapping hard and rapidly but when I looked at down, it was not moving (a slight hallucination). This caused me **a panic attack** because it felt so <u>very real</u>. I went to the bathroom and splashed cold water on my face and recovered from the delusion but it was very scary. The horrific bad trips other people have had when experimenting with drugs and getting high by other means, makes my experiences pale by comparison. **Drug abuse is a mistake on every level**, even when those who abuse them <u>believe they are in-control</u> and supposedly careful with their use.

Drugs used for the sake of 'a high' **are dangerous for lots of reasons**, bad trips being one of them.

Q & A: OPINION FIFTY-THREE

How Do Bipolar Sufferers Appear Emotionally?

A bipolar person will look <u>profoundly sad</u> at times and as if they are unable to enjoy their self.

They may also look **very tired and lacking in energy** and will often avoid being around other people. This is a description of their depressed phase.

In their mania phase, they will appear **very elated and happy**, to an exaggerated extent and they will seem to have an endless supply of energy at these times. They may also seem very creative at these times and want to work on projects endlessly or go on shopping sprees. They may also seem to be unable to relax and may avoid sleeping for days or even weeks at a time.

In-short, a bipolar person will appear extremely depressed, followed by episodes of appearing to be exaggeratedly happy. It is a mental illness, affecting the emotions and in repeating my previous description, has to do with extreme sadness, followed by exaggerated feelings of elation and happiness.

A personality disorder on the other hand (sometimes mistaken for bipolar disorder), has to do with **how one relates to other people** -- their treatment of them, and their reactions to them. This includes how they show affection toward people and whether or not they exercise manipulative type behaviors toward others. Some people have both emotional disorders and personality disorders **at the same time**.

Differences between OCD and Generalized Anxiety Disorder

With Obsessive Compulsive Disorder, there is usually an "acting out" aspect in which one repeats certain rituals having to do with daily tasks like washing their hands, turning off light switches, etc... These type things are **very strong impulses** with OCD sufferers because they feel they are not completing them thoroughly or completely enough. They may also obsess about something like germs getting on them and causing them illness and this will result in compulsive-avoidance behaviors, such as not wanting to touch other people and not wanting to go outside of their homes without gloves or something covering their mouth and nose to **prevent contracting germs**.

When repeated thoughts that one obsesses about, remain as simply thoughts, without the acting-out aspect, this would likely be more-so in the "Generalized Anxiety Disorder" category in which chronic thoughts of worry is a key manifestation. With GAD, people do worry and obsess about things like illness, school, work, relationships and yes, some GAD sufferers report struggling with their firmly held beliefs. This is not a psychosis but rather is in the "neurosis" category, so is not actually a mental illness per say, but rather a condition of chronic anxiety (thoughts of fear and worry).

I recommend that one does an online search, when in question about the differences between these disorders, using "OCD and GAD" as search terms and compare the descriptions of the two. I believe you will find that your compulsive worry and racing thoughts are more-so in the GAD category, due to your lack of the **acting-out aspect**. Also look into "Cognitive Behavioral Therapy" programs which are available online via a search as well and you can find coping though this type of therapy.

Q & A: OPINION FIFTY-FIVE

What other than Constipation causes Difficult Bowel Movements?

(Note: The digestive system is regulated by the INS.)

While IBS or another bowel disease is a possibility for **difficulty in having bowel movements**, one could also be suffering from a degree of bowel obstruction, meaning something in their large or small intestine is blocking the movement of fecal matter, into the lower part of the colon, where bowel movements can then occur.

Most blockages **are benign**, meaning not malignant (cancerous) and can include things like gallstones or pockets/pouches that form on the walls of the colon called "diverticula". These can be a quarter-inch or larger in diameter and if are found to be present in the colon via a "colonoscopy", a diagnosis of "Diverticulosis" would result (**"Diverticulitis"** is more severe).

This is another possibility for mild to severe obstruction of bowel movements and/or changes in the size and shape of them.

While it's relatively rare, especially if you are not age 50 or older, colon cancer can cause obstructed or small diameter bowel movements. More common causes can be things in your diet that cause thick consistency stools, meaning they become clay-like and sticky, so that it is more difficult to pass them because they stick to the sides of your colon. People who have to take iron supplements sometimes have this difficulty.

Other common causes can be bowel disorders such as IBS (Irritable Bowel Syndrome) as mentioned previously, Colitis, Celiac Disease (gluten intolerance) and Crohn's disease. These potentially cause **inflammation** in the intestines, causing them to swell and constrict. Simple constipation can cause thin or obstructed stools as well because part of the drier fecal matter stays in the colon while that which is less dry, passes through it when you have a bowel movement.

A medical physical would be important however, if for nothing else, to give one peace of mind, that it is not caused by something serious.

Q & A: OPINION FIFTY-SIX

Can Stress Aggravate the Symptoms of Chiari Malformation?

While I don't have Chiari Malformation, I do have autoimmune thyroid disease and neurological symptoms that I developed from long-term deficiencies in Vitamins D, E and B12. I find that stress can always **aggravate my symptoms**. Medical research studies have shown that stress can bring some diseases, such as autoimmune ones, to the surface and this has been specifically found to be true of Graves' disease.

It makes sense that this would be true of Chiari Malformation as well because it directly affects **the nervous system** and any neurological disorder can see flares of symptoms with added stressors. Even disorders like rheumatoid arthritis can be exacerbated by stress and **emotional overload**.

Also, when you settle down to rest and sleep, your body's metabolism slows to allow for relaxation and so that your body can repair any damaged cells that occur with daytime activities. This means the immune system and all of your organs are operating less-optimally in moderating things like fever and pain when you lack rest/sleep. They become inactive to **repair and replenishment**, when one is not getting proper rest. You also become still and inactive without proper rest and you are more finely tuned-into bodily sensations at these times, so that they seemingly become more amplified for this reason.

Q & A: OPINION FIFTY-SEVEN

Overcoming Social Phobia When Re-establishing a Relationship

Remind yourself through self-reassurance and repeating phrases to yourself, to the effect that even if you do get anxious in front of your re-established acquaintance, that **they will be understanding about it** and you will get past it without harming your relationship with them. You can also have a backup story handy, to inform them with, by simply saying you've been struggling a bit with added stressors (common with anxiety disorders) but that you know you'll get past it soon.

If they are a genuine friend, they will understand, if not and they are embarrassed or offended by your not immediately opening-up fully to them socially, you've lost nothing anyway (true friends should show understanding) and can move past them, onto better acquaintances. So you're suffering a bit of social phobia however, with time and effort, you can **learn to better cope with it**. Do a search online about "Cognitive Behavioral Therapy" and you'll find lots of good anxiety, self-help programs. None are very expensive and **some are offered free**.

Q & A: OPINION FIFTY-EIGHT

Are Antidepressants Overly-Prescribed?

The response that follows below, was to a post made by someone relating their story to me about their doctor prescribing them antidepressant drugs, later to be determined that they had medical conditions that were **delayed in being treated**. They asked my opinion as to whether I believed doctors were resorting too-often to the prescribing of psychiatric drugs as opposed to correct medical diagnoses. ----

It's hard to say what percent of doctors resort to prescribing abuse but my suspicion is that it is small. It does occur however and a doctor in my own city **lost his license to practice** over this very thing. I have to agree with you - that with endocrine disorders such as diabetes and thyroid diseases affecting so many tens of millions of people just in a country like the USA alone and with estimates stating that up to half who experience them are not being diagnosed, these should be tested for before **emotions-only diagnoses are made**.

Blood tests are so very diagnostic and are not that expensive, plus they only require a requisition by the doctor - so should be ordered for any patient who is experiencing emotional symptoms whether physical ones accompany them or not. This also being true with the fact that emotional symptoms of anxiety and depression are some of **the first that can manifest** with hyperthyroidism, hypothyroidism and hypoglycemia.

The same is true of <u>sex hormone imbalances</u> that can occur mostly with age or with adrenal gland problems that can occur mostly at any adult age.

One solution is for patients to **be proactive** in asking for tests to be ordered and in seeking a doctor willing to work with them in doing so. In some cases, a lack of diagnostic testing ordered by a doctor can also be due to a <u>lack of communication from patients,</u> who do not fully describe their symptoms as they should.

Q & A: OPINION FIFTY-NINE

Stomach Acid from GERD Entering the Lungs

There's very little available online as far as medical sources recommending what to do in the case of **stomach acid already entering the lungs**. I too have experienced this, actually choking several times and feeling the acid coming back up from my lungs into my throat when coughing (very strong burning sensation). My suspicion however is that <u>the body rids itself of the acid,</u> which is foreign in the lungs, by producing mucous and causing you to **cough it up**. This is also part of how it causes asthma symptoms. The acid also likely causes an <u>inflammatory reaction</u> which asthma sources state is part of why the passages narrow and tighten, plus produce extra mucous.

I also found over time with my own asthma that I experienced "orthopnea" - more difficult to breathe lying flat on my back - <u>supine</u>. This concerned me greatly at first but I found medical sources saying that orthopnea was **common with GERD** and some doctors speculate that the lungs begin to close when they sense the supine position to prevent more acid from entering them and causing further damage. As a precaution I asked my doctor for chest X-ray and a BNP blood test (one that detects heart enlargement) but both were negative. My BNP level in fact was very low at "4" - with normal being <100 (below 100).

An **elevated BNP** can mean <u>cardiac involvement</u> in asthma but it is actually rare if one is not elderly or has not experienced a heart attack or serious heart valve problems. I had the tests done more-so as **a precaution** and for <u>peace of mine</u>. NOTE: a BNP level of "100 to 300" indicates mild heart failure A level of "600 to 900" indicates moderate and a level of "900 and above" indicates severe heart failure/enlargement (The vast majority of asthma cases do not have cardiac involvement. Most cases are caused by allergies and GERD.)

I would say that if you feel acid go into your windpipe, to <u>purposefully induce a cough</u> until you feel you've rid your lungs of it, as best possible. Medical sources also recommend <u>elevating the head of your bed </u>by six inches by placing books or bricks under the headboard or front legs of it.

Also **taking an acid blocker** like Prilosec can help a great deal. It is important to see your doctor when acid reflux is severe, meaning chronic and ongoing, rather than occasional or mild in occurrence.

Q & A: OPINION SIXTY

What causes a Person to Experience Facial Swelling (Edema)?

(Note: Fluid regulation in the body and release of histamine by the immune system, are functions of the INS.)

With the swelling (edema) **being in your face**, it's possible that you're suffering from hypothyroidism - an under-active thyroid gland. Many times with hypothyroid conditions, swelling appears in the face.

In the old days of diagnosing it, they named it "myxedema" which actually means tissue swelling. Some thyroid patients see the swelling in other parts of their bodies as well, such as **feet and legs** and can occur with hyperthyroidism (overactive) as well.

Another possibility is sinus congestion or allergies to food, natural inhalants in your home (including pet dander) or an allergy to a makeup you are using.

Other less possible conditions would be nephrotic conditions causing edema, such as liver, heart or kidney disease but if these were the case, the swelling would show up in other parts of your body as well, **especially in the extremities**.

It is something worth having checked into by a doctor, to rule out serious causes and to get some treatment, such as an <u>antihistamine drug</u>.

SECTION FOUR:
Questions and Answers/Opinions 61 through 77

Q & A: OPINION SIXTY-ONE

I Take Four Types of Drugs – Which of Them Causes Edema (Swelling)?

(The four drugs I help define following below, was in response to someone asking questions about them, on a message board Q & A website, regarding which of them could cause fluid retention in the body.)

Amlodipine - is calcium channel blocker which can cause swelling as a side effect.

Armour Thyroid (the same brand I take for hypothyroidism) - is a natural thyroid hormone replacement drug and should not cause edema (swelling) but rather should help with any that is caused specifically **by hypothyroidism**.

Meloxicam - is a non-steroid but powerful anti-inflammatory drug but one side effect listed for it is **"swelling"**.

Hdrochlorothiazide - is a type of diuretic medication to help rid your body of fluid build-up, so should be helping with the swelling **rather than aggravating it**. It may be that your dose of this particular drug is not high enough but your doctor can help you to determine this.

You should inquire about it because high levels of fluid in the body can become dangerous if it begins **building in the lungs** and if you are not getting rid of it well enough through sufficient urinating, during the daytime and at night as well,if needed. The timing of your hdrochlorothiazide dose might also be an issue and if taken earlier might help you rid the fluid before lying down to sleep at night and being awakened frequently to urinate. This too can be determined by your doctor.

Q & A: OPINION SIXTY-TWO

Are There Self-Help Therapies for Anxiety Disorder?

One of the most effective therapies which can also be self-administered in addition to receiving it from a mental health professional is "**Cognitive Behavioral Therapy**" (CBT). This method helps one to react differently to emotions that tend to become imbalanced if reactions to them are not changed. It is a therapy that takes some time and practice but has a high treatment success rate. It also helps you to not fear the symptoms of strong emotion and to **change your behavior** in response to them, which over time diminishes their effects in hindering your ability to carry on normal life and activities. You also start to recognize these emotions as being natural in their proper context, so that you have less fear and dread of them.

In my opinion, CBT methods are the best available in learning to cope-with and possibly **completely overcome** anxiety and depression.

It worked for me tremendously well when I suffered severe anxiety symptoms and panic attacks from the onset of autoimmune thyroid disease and other co morbid health disorders I experienced.

One online source you might conduct a search on is the "National Association of Cognitive-Behavioral Therapists", which also gives updates on **CBT self-help programs they recommend**, as they become available. A general search on CBT will also yield you lots of helpful information.

Q & A: OPINION SIXTY-THREE

What causes Frequent Heavy Discharge?

(This was an actual question I replied-to on a Q & A message board website.) ---

It depends on from what part of the body the discharge comes from. If it comes from the vaginal area, it can vary and can be increased by <u>yeast infections</u> and <u>hormone imbalances,</u> both of which can be treated. If blood discharge becomes too heavy during menstrual cycles, this too needs medical attention because **it can cause anemia** if not treated.

Discharge from the nipples **can occur in women** as well, especially in those who are lactating (giving milk). When it occurs in women who aren't pregnant, it's called "Galactorrhea".

In most cases isn't of concern because it can be caused by certain prescribed drugs being taking or from irritation of the nipples, such as from wearing a particular garment or from being manipulated otherwise. A <u>rare cause</u> would be a **benign or malignant tumor.**

Men should not experience nipple discharge but if it occurs, this can indicate <u>severe hormone imbalance</u> or a tumor in the breast or in a regulating **endocrine gland.**

Anal discharge is not that uncommon in either men or women and is usually caused by a **bowel or digestive disorder** that either causes incontinence-diarrhea or mucous in the stool.

Q & A: OPINION SIXTY-FOUR

What Causes Red Itchy Hands and Right-Sided Stomach Pain?

The medical name for the itching and redness of the hands/palms is "**palmar erythema**" and there are a number of <u>possible causes</u> including nutritional deficiencies, pregnancy, some type of inflammation in the body and liver disease (i.e. hepatitis and cirrhosis). If there is also rash present, it might be a type of dermatitis.

With the possibility of liver involvement, especially with having the palm itching along with stomach pain you should definitely <u>see a doctor</u> for **further evaluation.**

If the redness on the skin includes whelps or blisters this would sound more like <u>severe hives</u> of some type or possibly even <u>Shingles</u> (herpes zoster), which can start as red spots and then progress to scabbing.

There are other less common possibilities, for hive type break-outs such as a type of Lupus that affects the skin called "**Discoid Lupus Erythematosus**" but my suspicion in your case (as you described in your post), is that it is a <u>more common</u> variety of hives.

With this type break-out, you should <u>see your doctor</u> for treatment and to rule out a cause that might result in more skin problems and scarring.

In regard to stomach pain in-general, a hernia of more than one possible type, is one possibility. Other things that are possible would be **ulcers or colitis** (when combined; "ulcerative colitis") and is also called "inflammatory bowel disease". A less concerning type of bowel problem is "irritable bowel syndrome" but with these bowel disorders/diseases, you should also be having either <u>constipation or diarrhea or both</u>.

Other less possible problems would be something like a **stomach aneurysm** (enlargement of an artery), a tumor or a problem in an organ such as the **liver or appendix**. I would say that it's definitely worth a trip to the doctor to have it investigated, if for nothing else, to give you peace of mind and <u>treatment recommendations</u>.

Q & A: OPINION SIXTY-FIVE

What are the BUN and Creatinine Blood Tests?

Those two blood tests are commonly ordered to evaluate a person's **kidney function** (an organ regulated by the INS) but they can also be used to monitor for other types of disease and disorders.

The "BUN" test stands for "Blood Urea Nitrogen" and both it and "creatinine" can help to determine how well the kidneys are **filtering-out waste products and toxins** from the blood. If either or both are elevated, this can indicate kidney dysfunction (failure for the kidneys to remove all of these substances from the blood).

The "Albumin" test is more often one ordered to evaluate liver function but may be ordered in combination with the BUN and creatinine level due to the fact that with liver dysfunction, **waste products and toxins** can also build in the blood, to a degree that the kidneys are unable to filter them out completely. In the case of Albumin, liver disease may be present **if the level is low** (below normal) rather than elevated.

Two other blood tests of liver function are these liver enzymes:

ALT - Alanine AminoTransferase

AST (SGOT) - Aspartate AminoTransferase/Serum Glutamic Oxaloacetic Transaminase

<u>Q & A: OPINION SIXTY-SIX</u>

What is the Significance of a Blood Creatinine Level?

Different labs have different ranges and some use a decimal point for the blood measurement of creatinine while others may not. A <u>low creatinine</u> is not common and not usually indicative of a problem, other than <u>possible loss of muscle mass</u> and I will attempt to explain how the blood levels react to muscle changes and or changes in kidney function, following.

Creatinine is a substance that is **released into the blood stream by muscle tissue** in the body and it is normal to have a level of it in the blood at all times because muscle tissue continually <u>breaks down and regenerates</u> in the body throughout one's lifetime. The level however should be in the normal range for one's age. The level can go down in the elderly due to their <u>natural loss of muscle tone</u> but it can go down in level due to inadequate muscle content in the body for other reasons as well, such as in **diseases that cause muscle atrophy** (loss). When muscles are injured or damaged, a temporary increase in creatinine can result.

One of the jobs of the kidneys is to <u>clear any excess creatinine from the blood stream</u> so that it is flushed out of the body through the urine. If the level rises, this can be due to malfunction in one or both of a person's kidneys, due to a disease within them or **kidney stones**.

Some men with **prostrate gland problems** can see an increase in creatinine as well if it causes urinating dysfunction or infrequency. Diabetes can cause damage to the kidneys as well, as can prolonged hypertension and these can raise the level as well.

A **low creatinine**, in my opinion is of much less concern than would be an **elevated level**.

Q & A: OPINION SIXTY-SEVEN

If I Stop my Medication for Bipolar what Happens?

With bipolar disorder, the two emotions that manifest are extreme depression alternating with spells of mania or what might also be seen as an exaggerated elation. Medication for bipolar helps to level-out these two opposite poles so that the person doesn't experience the extreme peaks and valleys but is on **a more even plane** with their emotions. The poles in-essence come closer together rather than being so far apart.

When a bipolar patients stops taking their medication, these poles begin to spread apart again, so that **extreme opposites in emotion are experienced**, as occurs in diagnosed patients, before treatment. This will result in times of withdrawal from others, profound sadness, lack of energy and the need to sleep excessively. This would also include the inability to enjoy things that once brought pleasure (major, severe depression).

This will be followed by times of the person <u>feeling highly energetic</u>, with erratic behaviors being displayed, inability to sleep during these times, sprees of shopping or working on projects endlessly (manic episodes).

It is very important that bipolar patients not to stop their drug therapies because they can actually **experience a worsening** of these extremes of emotion when the leveling effect of the medication is <u>suddenly halted</u>. This is why some patients who stop their drugs 'cold turkey', display bizarre behaviors or develop suicidal or violent tendencies.

<u>Q & A: OPINION SIXTY-EIGHT</u>

What are some Common Causes of Fatigue in Women?

(The response below was to a question asked by a middle-aged female, with <u>fatigue symptoms</u> but who had a normal CBC test.)

In my opinion, women with symptoms like yours should be more thoroughly evaluated, if a complete blood count like you've already had done, doesn't reveal a cause. You should also have blood tests of your **sex and adrenal hormones** ordered, to see if they are imbalanced, such as that which occurs with **menopause and perimenopause** (pre-menopause) and with conditions like <u>PECOS</u> ("Polycystic Ovary Syndrome").

You should also have a **fasting glucose level ordered** to check for diabetes and a thyroid panel to check for hypothyroid or hyperthyroid disorders. The major vitamins such as B12 and the D level might also need ordered. These tests might zero-in on a problem that is responsible for your symptoms or at least **rule them out**, so that even further evaluation can be undertaken if needed.

Q & A: OPINION SIXTY-NINE

Is Osgood-Schlatter Disease an Arthritic Condition?

With Osgood-Schlatter disease the tendon that lies between the top of the shin bone and the bottom of the thigh bone - connecting the quadricep muscle to the shin-bone, becomes inflamed from being **excessively stretched** as it works the thigh muscle with the bending of the knee joint ("tendonitis"). This also inflames and irritates the nerves in the area of the joint and muscles. As the tendon becomes inflamed, it may also cause a bump that can be seen on the outside - bottom part of the knee (a nodule), that is painful when pressed-on. It can also cause edema around the knee (swelling).

Athletes and people who work jobs that require **a great deal of knee movement**, can develop Osgood-Schlatter disease but it can be treated by putting ice packs on and around the knee to reduce swelling and by taking an over-the-counter or prescription anti-inflammatory drug (depending on severity), for pain.

Keeping the knee joint inactive for as long as possible (isolated) can also help the tendonitis, as can gentle message and slow, **low-impact stretching exercises** to keep the joint from stiffening.

Q & A: OPINION SEVENTY

Is There an Effective Method for Coping with Panic Attacks?

One method that some former panic attack sufferers have used is to **not resist them** but to actually invite them to occur. While this sounds strange at first glance, it is a method that in-essence tricks the "fight or flight response" into reversing itself. This **anxiety mechanism** thrives on resistance and fear; in fact these are triggers for panic attacks. By literally **challenging anxiety** to takes its best shot, you cause it to shut down because the fuel (fearful anticipation) is not there for anxiety to run on.

Part of this method can also involve learning to flow with anxiety, so that you work with it, rather than it working against you. By practicing this aspect, one can eventually learn to **channel anxiety** into a positive direction, such as toward a creative process (i.e. art, sports, writing, etc...).

One PhD psychiatrist in the UK discovered that by having patients **conjure-up torrid romantic fantasies** in their minds, they could stop anxiety and panic attacks in their tracks.

Again, this is <u>an unusual method</u> but one that the doctor's patients found relief from anxiety by practicing. This would be more-so in the "diversion method" category and one that other psychiatrists have found effective in different versions for many years.

"Exposure therapy" is a method in which an anxiety sufferer exposes their self to those **things that trigger their phobias**. They do so <u>gradually</u> until the fear comes under their control and that sometimes completely subsides for them over time.

These methods take <u>time and effort</u> but can be effective in overcoming anxiety and panic attacks. It can also help to **join anxiety forums** and read/share <u>personal anxiety experiences</u> and <u>coping-gains</u> with fellow sufferers.

<u>Q & A: OPINION SEVENTY-ONE</u>

Are Liver ALT and AST Levels in the 100s Significant?

(The question I responded-to below, was posted by someone on behalf of their daughter.)

Yes, possibly <u>too high</u> to be simply a fatty liver problem. They should also blood test her "Alkaline Phosphatase" level, the "Gamma-Glutamyl Transpeptidase" (GGT) and her bilirubin level. These three liver function tests **can help better evaluate** what may be causing her liver enzyme, elevation problem.

These tests for example, can help determine if she might have a gallstone obstructing her bile duct in the liver or if the bile duct is diseased for some reason. Some medications and drugs can cause high liver enzyme levels in susceptible people and of course things like **alcohol abuse** can as well. There are also a number of types of hepatitis as well and there are specific tests that will detect them.

A more **thorough evaluation** ASAP is very important with elevations of ALT and AST that high (in the 100s) or an elevation that is that high on any other liver function test for that matter.

Q & A: OPINION SEVENTY-TWO

How Do People Develop Social Anxiety Disorder?

Some anxiety research groups believe that **social phobia** often begins in childhood and progresses as a person enters adulthood. The sympathetic nervous system response called "the fight or flight response" begins to trigger inappropriately. Like other anxiety disorders, the negative responses a person has to feeling anxious about **social events or settings** they are attending or planning to attend (immediate or anticipated anxiety), becomes more of a learned behavior. A person with Social Anxiety Disorder (SAD) for example, may experience panic attacks when socializing with one or more people that they do not already know well.

They may **avoid social settings** because of their uncomfortable anxiety symptoms when around people. These reactions cause the anxiety disorder to worsen and it will eventually many times, need drug and/or psychiatric therapy, for coping to occur, or to even overcome the anxiety of socializing, over time.

People with SAD, develop **fears of being judged by others** whom they believe to be observing them closely, as to how well they converse with others and as to how well they display their social mannerisms. In reality, others are not observing them as closely as they think they are and these people are usually more comfortable around them than they believe they are. It is a type of **extreme or exaggerated shyness** that can seriously affect quality of life and the ability to cope in society. Sad can restrict a person's life so that they do not want to go out into the public for any reason, including things like shopping for food or going to the post office, to a doctor visit, etc...

Entertainer - Donny Osmond is one famous sufferer of social phobia, with associated panic attacks that he attests to being present **beginning in his childhood**. He has however, learned to cope with SAD, through drug therapy and Cognitive Behavioral Therapy and he has since **served as a spokesman** for people with anxiety disorders.

Q & A: OPINION SEVENTY-THREE

What is a Simple Description of Asthma?

Asthma is an inflammatory disease of the lung passages (bronchial tubes), in which they begin to narrow and produce a thick, sticky mucous that causes **wheezing and coughing**, especially after exercise. Many asthma patients have worse symptoms at night and early morning and some have more difficulty breathing in the supine position (when lying down flat of their backs).

The vast majority of asthma cases are caused by allergies to things being inhaled from the air when taking-in oxygen, such as dust, pollen and pet dander. A more rare cause of asthma, is **congestive heart failure**, in which a person with heart disease develops an enlarged heart, causing large amounts of fluid to build in the lungs, due to release of a hormone by the kidneys (BNP), that responds to the stretching of the heart muscle. This type called "cardiac asthma" however is more common in heart disease, patients, and the elderly and in people with serious heart defects and represents **a very small percent of cases**, when compared to the much more common allergic asthma.

Also: Both asthma and GERD have potential to cause anxiety symptoms and those of worry but your doctor can suggest something to help you in this area as well if you find any difficulty coping.

There are self help psychiatric therapies as well, such as Cognitive Behavioral Therapy that can help one deal with negative emotions caused by asthma or other physical illnesses. I used such methods when I was dealing with symptoms of thyroid disease and found them to be very effective.

Q & A: OPINION SEVENTY-FOUR

Can Getting Ample Sunlight Still Leave You Vitamin D Deficient?

(Note: The body absorbs vitamins through the diet, by way of the digestive system and through the skin via activation by sunlight, which are responses regulated by the INS.)

You can still be low on vitamin D, **even with getting plenty of sunshine** because much of what the body needs also comes through the diet and while many foods have vitamin D in them, a person can fail to absorb it, due to **digestive problems.** People with autoimmune gastro-intestinal disorders, such as Crohn's Disease, Celiac Disease and Pernicious Anemia, can have problems absorbing vitamins from things in their diets because they lack the **intestinal enzymes** that are needed to do so, due to them being destroyed by auto-antibodies that **come from the immune system.**

Chronic diarrhea, that occurs for any reason can also cause failure to absorb vitamins such as D and the other major nutrients. A condition called "malabsorption syndrome" can as well and this one occurs due to gallstones obstructing the bile duct that goes from the gallbladder to the liver or from the duct being destroyed by an autoimmune process (biliary cirrhosis). The malabsorption can also be due to a person not being able to **absorb fat from the diet** (fat malabsorption syndrome) and since some vitamins, such as D, E, A and K are "fat soluble", if fat is not properly absorbed from the diet, the vitamins have no carrier substance to take them into the cells of the body.

For these reasons, adequate amounts of sunshine **may still not be enough** to prevent vitamin D deficiency and when it occurs, **high-dose oral supplementation is required** to get levels back to normal range and afterward, the highest RDA of vitamin D will likely be required for the rest of one's life.

Q & A: OPINION SEVENTY-FIVE

Are Fluttering Heart Beats Dangerous?

The heart rate is regulated by electrical impulses supplied by the nervous system to stimulate each beat and **the number of beats** with different levels of physical activity. Heart flutters are a type of palpitation, meaning you are aware of the strange beating because you can feel it.

They are usually a <u>benign</u> (not dangerous) type of temporary, **intermittent arrhythmia** that only lasts a few seconds at the most, although some people experience them many times in a day or continuously. The type of arrhythmias that are of more concern, are those that occur for <u>sustained amounts of time</u>, such as for several minutes, hours or even days and they are in the "atrial fibrillation" or "atrial flutter" categories.

Sometimes, instead of a flutter, people will feel **an extra beat**, <u>a skipped beat</u> or one that seems **extra hard** (a very noticeable thump) and these are called "premature ventricular contractions" (PVCs) and while these can also indicate a health problem, they **most often are benign** and occur in people without any heart or blood pressure problems, including young people.

Either type of heart palpitation is still worthy of discussing with your doctor, <u>as a precaution</u> and to give you peace of mind, that **a serious condition is not present**. As stated in previous posts I have made in regard to heart murmurs, caffeine and other stimulants, including alcohol <u>can aggravate these palpitations</u> in some people, as can <u>stress and anxiety</u>.

Some people also have a common heart murmur than can contribute to palpitations called "Mitral Valve Prolapse" (MVP) but this too is **a benign heart condition** in the vast majority of cases and does not pose a real danger, despite the sometimes concerning symptoms it can cause.

Some medical sources state that MVP affects **up to 20% of the population** and can manifest with spells of tachycardia (rapid heartbeat) and it can also cause mild chest pain and discomfort. It also causes anxiety symptoms commonly but there's a possibility that you have anxiety causing heart palpitations, without MVP being present.

Other possibilities for anxiety symptoms and tachycardia would be **episodes of hypoglycemia** (low blood glucose) and while this is misunderstood by much of the public, low blood sugar causes adrenaline surges and can occur without diabetes being present, which is referred-to as "reactive hypoglycemia". You might also be suffering an electrolyte imbalance of sodium, potassium, magnesium, etc...

A medical physical and blood testing might be necessary **to find the cause** if it doesn't become evident without these.

Q & A: OPINION SEVENTY-SIX

What causes Flashes and Twinkles of Light in my Peripheral Vision?

(Note: Eyesight is made possible via cranial and optic nerves and nerve-fibers.)

My suspicion is that you are referring to lights appearing that are **really not there** but appear to be real.

It's funny you mention this because I have at times experienced seeing a light to the side of my vision, when my eyes are closed. In my case, the light actually seems to dance around a bit (flickers and changes position). I also experience occasional **star-type lights** that appear for just a second or two and then are gone and these can be a different color each time it happens - sometime red, blue or green. This star twinkle experience happens to a lot of people because I've posted on forums in the past on which several members would admit to this eyesight phenomenon happening to them. Who knows what the lights are but they could simply be **neurotransmitters firing in the brain** or maybe they are something spiritual (our guardian angels winking at us perhaps).

Rarely, seeing lights can be a sign of neurological problems, including MS (multiple sclerosis) but not if they are stand-alone symptoms and you're not also having numbness in your limbs or symptoms of peripheral neuropathy (tingling, stabbing or numbness in hands or feet). One other possibility is that you have a slightly injured blood vessel in your eye but **an optometrist**, could exam you and tell you **if that is the case.** My dad had a blood vessel to rupture in his eye but it was originally injured when he was a child and he saw what he described as shooting stars that constantly flew across the field of his vision.

These are possibilities but even your regular MD can likely **rule out anything serious** with a hand held ophthalmoscope, which shines a light into your eyeball. An optometrist can also do this, with a more sophisticated ophthalmoscope evaluation, to make sure you don't have glaucoma present or "choroidal nevus"(small eye tumor), both of which can **potentially cause lights in your vision.**

Q & A: OPINION SEVENTY-SEVEN

Why is my Heart Rate 120 Beats-Per-Minute at Rest?

Medical sources state that tachycardia (rapid heart rate) is recognized when the beats per minute at rest are at **100 BPM or more**, so yours is tachycardia but not as severe as some people attest to experiencing. I've seen people report a continuous resting heart rate that never goes below 140 or 150 and is sometimes at 200 BPM! Regardless, yours is something to be further evaluated for cause and may be something simple and benign (not threatening) and fairly **easily fixed.**

Some things that come to mind would be hormone or nutritional imbalances. Elevated thyroid hormone levels for example (hyperthyroidism) can result in sustained or intermittent spells of tachycardia, as can imbalances in essential **electrolytes in the blood,** such as low magnesium.

There is also a common heart murmur called "Mitral Valve Prolapse" that can cause **spells of tachycardia** but in most people it is not a life or health threatening condition, although symptoms from it can be life-disrupting.

Hormone imbalances, whether thyroid, adrenal, glucose-related or sex ones, can all be **brought back to balance** and so can electrolyte imbalances if they are present. Mitral Valve Prolapse, if causing symptoms of heart palpitations can be fixed in many cases, simply with **low-dose beta-blocker drugs**.

Your cardiologist will better evaluate your case and I'm willing to bet that he or she will be able to fix your tachycardia and I send my best wishes and hopes to you, for a simple solution!

(END)